Contents

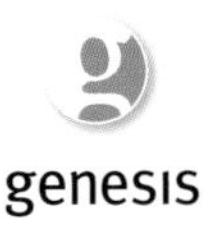

This edition published 2009 by Genesis Publishing

8, Neptune Court, Vanguard Way
Ocean Park, Cardiff CF24 5PJ

A CIP catalogue record for this book is available from the British Library.

ISBN: 978-0-9564285-0-9

www.genesispublishing.co.uk

Introduction

We all love it when people say, "You're looking well". It's even better when they say, "Wow, what happened to all that weight?"

Some of us have to work hard to keep in trim. Others are fortunate enough to look slim and well most, if not all of the time. I was one of those lucky ones for most of my life. Then, as for many of us, middle age happened to me. I ballooned up in weight, lost any fitness I had to start with (which wasn't that much, granted!), and found myself eating all the wrong things.

Then, like 2.6 million of us in the UK alone, I discovered that I had diabetes.

It's a familiar story. It might even be your story too, or that of someone you love. The road back to good health can look long and daunting. The prospect of cutting back on the foods that you love... of having to start exercising... it's not everyone's cup of herbal tea!

But I'd like to offer you some hope.

In six months I shed four stone. I found a diet that I really enjoyed. And I discovered the satisfaction – of not only being able to exercise, but actually enjoying it too.

But the biggest achievement of all was to reverse my diabetes.

Doctors may tell you that diabetes is incurable.

That once you have it, you'll always have it. Well yes, but what has happened to me is that I no longer have the symptoms, I can eat and drink (within reasonable limits) what I want. And I don't HAVE to get on the treadmill every day either!

My body is back under control. My control. And my life is back in balance – and I hope that, with the help of this book, yours will soon be too.

In fact, it's worth mentioning that writing this book was never my idea. When I guested on a BBC Radio Wales show with hosts Jamie and Louise, to talk about how I had reversed my diabetes, Jamie Owen (no relation!) urged me to share my story with more people in the form of a short book. And everywhere I go – not just in this country, but as part of my work in the States, the Middle East - people ask me to tell them how it can be done.

Some are diabetic themselves, or have friends and relatives who are. Some just want to lose weight – fast! This book is for all of you!

If it reassures you, my first attempt at losing weight didn't succeed. Nor the second one. Or, if I'm honest, the third one either. But what I learned during those failed attempts helped me fine-tune the method that you'll find set out in this book, an approach that anyone can have a go at – whether you're 15 or 75, clinically obese or just sporting a few extra inches of waistline.

I came to realise that some aspects of the diets I had been trying were working. But something about each of them meant that I kept slipping off them, or that the progress I was making went so far... but not as far as I wanted. The answer was to look at the science behind what I was doing, and also at my own tastes and lifestyle, and create a diet that worked for me. If you have tried a lot of different diets, you may find some aspects familiar – but not in the combination you see here.

And before you sit there and imagine the pounds evaporating, let me tell you that you will need a degree of willpower – and also a genuine desire to change the way you look and feel. Just as it is virtually impossible to give up smoking if you are only half-hearted about it, no diet will work if part of you insists on reaching for the crisps and chips when you feel peckish.

But why this diet – above all the others I have tried – has a good chance of working, is that you won't feel as hungry as you do on so many of them. And you get to eat really nice, filling food – so satisfying two of the biggest reasons why we eat: for comfort and for pleasure.

Yes, it will involve you making some changes to the way you shop and cook. But having looked at (and tried!) some of the other diets, I know this is a really tasty and enjoyable way to lose weight. And it doesn't involve buying any expensive specially made products either – just good, healthy ingredients you will find in any supermarket.

There is also some leeway to allow for people with different tastes than mine, and for when certain ingredients are out of season and unduly expensive.

In fact, just to keep you reading past the next few chapters, let me tell you one wonderful fact about this diet: it allows you to eat five times a day. Yes, five. And not hamster food either. But delicious fish, meat and even chocolate. You can even eat out on this diet. Later in the book I set out the things on a Chinese or Indian menu that will let you keep going to your favourite takeaway.

Losing weight, getting back into shape and looking good can only partly be achieved by eating the right foods. What I have done has also been achieved, in part, by adopting an exercise regime that has boosted my metabolism, improved the way my body's insulin functions, really accelerated my weight loss and put my heart, lungs and body in better shape. And while you'll find pictures of me proudly finishing a half marathon, don't panic. You won't have to do the same! I did my long runs well after I had lost four stone and reversed my diabetes.

Taking part in that run, in large part, was me proving to myself that I really could go all the way – and a celebration of regaining control of my body.

But if you are serious about getting your body – and possibly your diabetes too, if you are suffering from that -

back under your control, I would seriously suggest you incorporate exercise in your lifestyle. It doesn't have to be anything too strenuous. I achieved my weight loss having an enjoyable time in the health club and without ever breaking into a serious sweat. You can too.

My life has been turned around with this diet and exercise regime and I want to share it with you. Why? Because this isn't some miracle cure that relies on unproven (and unprovable) science. It's based on solid fact. It is really, really do-able.

It's all about giving your body the food it needs to get through a busy day, so you won't be gripping your tummy with hunger pangs, but training it to stop wanting the wrong foods that pile on the weight.

What's more, this is not a diet that is written in stone. Within some reasonable boundaries, you can adapt it to suit your own lifestyle, budget and tastebuds. I'll tell you how it worked for me, and it's up to you to either follow it down to the letter, or use the basics that I set out and modify it. After all, we are all different people, enjoy different things and our bodies work in different ways.

But above all, you will need to get your mind around one thing: you must enjoy your diet and not 'suffer with it'. You do that by letting your body know who is in control: you or the junk food that is wrecking your health.

And yes, much of the food we eat IS junk food. It's stuffed

with processed carbohydrates that do us as much harm as good. Even many so-called health foods contain sugars that we don't really need. Understanding why certain foods pile on weight while others give us a ready and steady supply of energy is one of the biggest steps to regaining control of your body – and I go through that in this book too. Knowing what you're eating really is a key step to enjoying what you're eating.

Enjoy a diet? I can hear you saying. Yes, enjoy it. Take a look at the recipes in the back of this book and tell me that they aren't delicious – and generous. And you'll be eating five times a day – which can't be bad! The secret is in reducing the amount of sugar you put into your body. No, not just the stuff you put in your tea and which is pumped into so many of our processed foods. But the natural sugars that so many of even our natural foods contain.

If a lot of what I'm writing about sounds familiar, that's because the starting point of me losing weight, beating my diabetes – and possibly saving my life - was an excellent book called 'The South Beach Diet' by cardiologist Dr Arthur Agatston. His book – dedicated to countering heart problems and diabetes - is based on cutting back on the foods that cause a rapid rise in blood sugar, the ones with a high GI level, and he goes into chapter and verse on how they impact upon your body. It is highly recommended reading.

I have taken the basic premise of his work – that there are 'good carbs' and 'bad carbs', as well as 'good fats' and 'bad fats' – and if you cut out the bad stuff, you can still eat well. I did, and then developed a diet using many of his basic premises (the ones that suited me!) and adapting my own version of it.

My diet is also based on what I call my 'famous five' – four 'green' and one 'red' foods – which not only provide the energy you need to get through a day without feeling hungry, but which will also contribute towards the 'detox' process necessary if you are going to change your longings for certain foods. What's more, you can eat as much of these 'famous five' foods as you wish!

I also want to let you know that this is a diet that you can follow regardless of how busy your life is. My life is as hectic as anyone's that I know. I rush from meeting to meeting and from event to event. But the recipes are so simple that a little thought and preparation means that many of your meals can be prepared in advance, and the rest take just minutes.

So are you ready to change your life? First I'll tell you how it happened for me – to show you how easy it could be for you too.

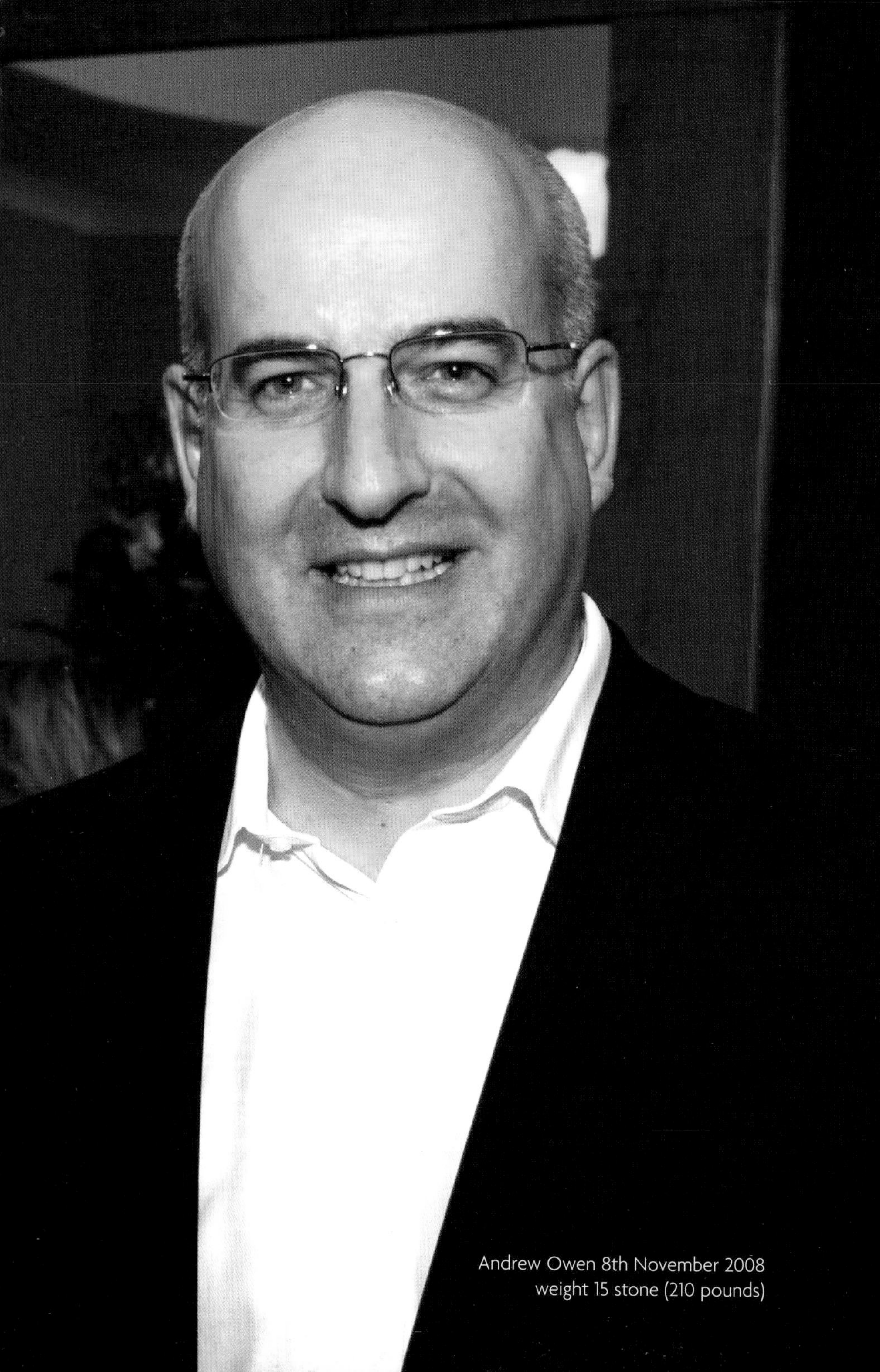

Andrew Owen 8th November 2008
weight 15 stone (210 pounds)

Chapter 1
The diagnosis

"Now I was starting to worry. I didn't know too much about blood sugar – and I wasn't off the scale with those two readings. But I do know that high levels of cholesterol can mean heart problems. I could only assume it was to do with the way I ate – and what I ate. The memories of all those late night curries came dancing before my mind's eye".

"Andrew! Thanks for coming in. I thought it was better if we could talk about your results rather than me writing to you or phoning you up."

This sounded a bit ominous. All I'd done was to go to my doctor's surgery and have a few tests carried out to keep my life insurance company happy. Just routine they said. And here I was being summoned back to my doctor for the results.

"Andrew, how have you been feeling lately?" she said, looking at me over the results in front of her.

"Umm, well not great if I'm honest. Been under the cosh at work lately, even more than usual, so a bit stressed and tired I suppose. But nothing very different from how I often feel. I've been taking the blood pressure tablets you've been giving me, so I'm guessing that's under control. No major aches or pains. Why?"

"It's these results from your blood tests. Your blood can tell you a lot about your general health, of course, and these show that you've got a blood sugar level of 6.7."

"What's a good level?" I asked, starting to worry now.

"Not what you have!" said the doctor. "But what's particularly worrying is what we call your 'fasting glucose level' – that's how much glucose you have in your blood before you have any food in the morning. It's the point in the day when you should be hungry, and your glucose levels should be relatively low. That was at 6.9. I'd have been a lot happier if it had been a bit closer to 6. It means that your body isn't processing glucose properly. Which points to a problem with your pancreas.

"The urine sample we took also showed a very high level of sugars. Far higher than you should expect to see. Again, that means that your body isn't processing the energy you're putting into it in the form of food.

"Then you have a cholesterol level of 8.3 and that is worrying. Ideally you'd be below 5.7. In fact, anything over 7.8 is regarded as 'very high'."

Now I was starting to worry. I didn't know too much about blood sugar – and I wasn't off the scale with those two readings. But I do know that high levels of cholesterol can mean heart problems. I could only assume it was to do with the way I ate – and what I ate. The memories of all those late night curries came dancing before my mind's eye.

But couldn't they give you tablets to fix cholesterol? Statins, I seemed to remember. I was probably going to get a ticking off, told to mend my ways and trim the waistline a bit. Then she'd pack me off with a prescription or two. For someone just into their forties, I couldn't be that unusual. There must be thousands of guys like me in a similar position. I had already been on blood pressure tablets for four or five years – and that had kept my condition in check. This was just a stage on – wasn't it?

"Is that it, doc? No more bad news is there?"

"Um, have you ever heard of 'triglycerides'?"

"No – are they good or bad?

"Well, like a lot of things, it depends on how many of them you have in your blood. They're a type of fat. Basically, if your body can't use up all the energy you make from the food you eat, the 'leftovers' get turned into triglycerides. And they can then get laid down as fatty deposits. Bad for your heart, your kidneys... need I go on?"

"And how I am doing in the 'tri-thingey, leftover fat' stakes?"

"Well a raised blood triglyceride level is 1.7 millimoles per litre. And yours is... 11.4. That isn't just bad. It's downright dangerous."

"But I can take medicine for all this, right, Doc?"

"Well yes you can. They should stabilise some of the most dangerous levels, and I've made out your first prescription here. I'd better tell you what they are, because you could be on them for some time.

"Aspirin you'll know all about, but it's not to help with a headache – although you've probably got one now. It's there to help prevent blood clots. Losartan – that's for your blood pressure. Atenolol – or what you'd probably call a 'beta blocker'. And Simvastatin – that's a statin to you. So hopefully between that lot, you might end up rattling when you walk, but we can get your cholesterol and triglyceride levels down and keep your blood pressure at a sensible level too."

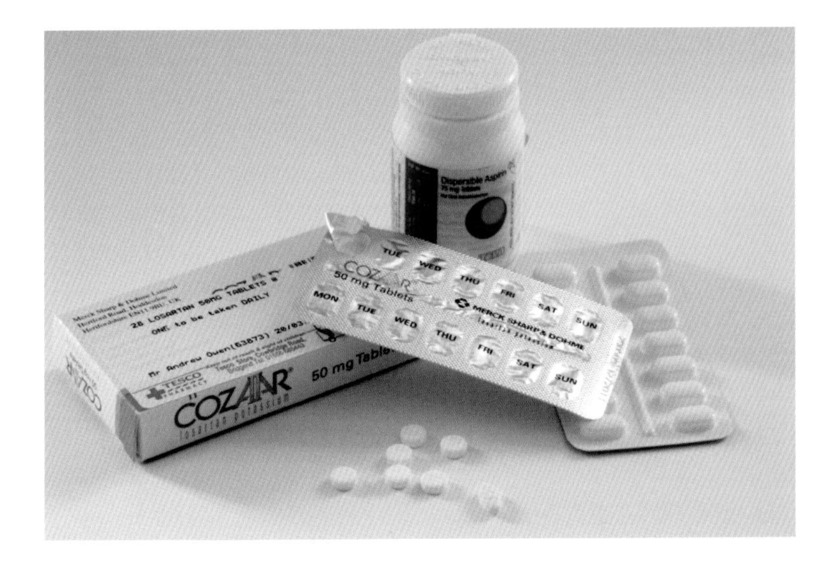

Just like I thought. A ticking off and a bunch of tablets. Except...

"But there's another underlying condition which won't be as easy to sort out. I'm afraid you have Type 2 diabetes."

This check up for my life insurance company was not going well. What else was she going to tell me? And why didn't I realise before that I had diabetes? That always sounded pretty heavyweight to me.

"I thought that was really dangerous unless it was treated, Doctor."

"It certainly can be. But there are many, many people in this country walking about with diabetes without knowing it. Millions more have 'pre-diabetes' – the high blood sugar level which is often a pre-cursor to full blown diabetes. If they're lucky, they will go to their doctor's with another problem and present symptoms which lead to a diagnosis. Like feeling tired and thirsty all the time. Or they get a check up like you did. The unlucky ones can lose their eyesight – or even die – before they realise they have diabetes.

"You're a very fortunate man, Andrew!"

I didn't feel it. I had sky-high levels of dangerous fats in my body, and Type 2 Diabetes. But at least I knew what I had. "I can fight this, right Doc? I can diet, exercise, get better, yes?"

"You'll have to diet, I'd also recommend a moderate exercise regime. Looking at you, you could usefully shed three stone. And yes, if you do that you'll start to feel better. But you've got diabetes now. That won't go away. Ever. You have to learn to live with it."

How wrong she was.

Chapter 2
I find out more about my condition

"Some 2.5 million people in the UK alone have diabetes, two million of them Type 2. A truly staggering figure out of a population of just over 60 million. And, as my doctor told me, half a million of those people don't even realise they have it. They are, literally, a ticking time-bomb."

Some people prefer not to know too many of the gory details about their condition. Others need to know everything. I'm one of those people. To me, finding out what had happened to my body while I thought I was just getting on with my life was the first stage to getting it back on track.

What I found out staggered me, quite frankly. I knew a lot of people were suffering from diabetes, and that the problem is getting worse, but I had no idea of the scale of it. We're always being told that the developed world is actually in the middle of an 'obesity epidemic'. You just have to look around you to see that – and those are the people you see because they're out, going to work or shopping. There are many, many more who rarely leave the house because they find it emotionally, or even physically difficult, to do so.

Only very recently, the world's fattest man was identified as someone living in Ipswich – all 70 stone of him. It's not just an American problem! Of course one of the biggest side effects of all that overeating and sitting in front of the TV is diabetes. The World Health Organisation reckons that over 180 million people round the world have diabetes – most of them the Type 2 diabetes which I was diagnosed with.

The two types of diabetes are quite different from each other. Type 1 diabetes is less common than Type 2, you cannot prevent it from happening and it develops when the body stops being able to produce insulin; it also usually appears before the age of 40.

Type 2, in contrast, is usually something that happens because of your lifestyle. It used to be known as 'adult-onset' diabetes - because it normally hits people later in life after years of poor diet and lack of exercise. Not any more. It's now rife amongst young adults and even children, which tells you all you need to know about what we are doing with our bodies in today's society. Look around the supermarket and see just how many of the 'special offers', 'BOGOFs' and 'two for ones' are not the healthy foods, but the fatty, calorie-rich, processed foods.

Those on lower incomes will often be tempted to buy these offers because they're a cheap way to fill up their family, and the recession is not helping either. Walk through a supermarket and judge for yourself how many aisles are taken up with crisps, sweets, processed breads, biscuits and snacks – and compare it to the space given over to fresh vegetables and fruit...

When I was young, a couple of kids in each class might be overweight. Today, it can be a really high proportion. Each child, on average, is nine pounds heavier than 20 years ago. A tenth of children are categorised as 'clinically obese'. No wonder they say that this might be the first generation that doesn't live as long as their parents. A survey came out in October 2009 that showed, for the first time, that more than half of us are 'overweight' or 'obese'.

A quarter of us are actually obese. And 'obese' doesn't mean cuddly. It means we are carrying weight that will shorten our lives. The annual NHS bill for diabetes alone is £600 million.

It's hardly surprising when you look at the differences between the way we live now and even 30 or 40 years ago. Then, many people had their own allotment and so had a regular supply of free vegetables; and doing the shopping meant going (usually walking) to the butchers, bakers, greengrocers and corner shop for their food... not getting into the car and piling up the trolley at the supermarket once a week.

On top of that, if you wanted to get to school or work it invariably meant walking at least part of the way – and work itself was more physical than it is today.

We've become a nation of 'snackers' or 'browsers' between our meals and when we sit and watch TV. It's a chilling thought that if you eat just 200 calories a day more than you need – that's pretty much a regular packet of crisps – you will pile on a stone and a half over 12 months. Popping into your nearest coffee shop for a full milk latte every day as a pick-me-up could have the same effect.

It's so easy to consume more calories than you use – not least because it's so hard to know how many calories you're taking on board. One of the outcomes is that some 2.5 million people in the UK alone have diabetes, two million of them Type 2. A truly staggering figure out of a population of just over 60 million. And, as my doctor told me, half a million of those people don't even realise they have it. They are, literally, a ticking time-bomb.

Being overweight isn't the only cause of Type 2 diabetes -

but it's a very common starting point because it involves a sustained history of eating and drinking more than we need – and putting our bodies under pressure to cope with all that extra load. Essentially, Type 2 or 'Diabetes mellitus' is a condition where the amount of glucose in the blood is too high because the body cannot use it properly.

We get our glucose from the digestion of food and drinks containing carbohydrate, and it is also produced by the liver. Most of us think of carbohydrates as starchy foods such as bread, potatoes, pasta and chapattis, but it also comes from fruit, dairy products, sugar and other sweet foods. It's food that fuels us – but a car will only use the petrol it needs to get from A to B. Our bodies are the same.

The real problems for the body start when all that extra food we have pumped into us continually overloads our system so it can't make enough insulin to cope with all the glucose we are generating. Insulin is the hormone produced by our pancreas which 'unlocks the door' and helps the glucose to enter the cells where it is then used as fuel for energy. Problems can also occur when the insulin that is produced does not work properly (that is also known as insulin resistance). In most (but not all) cases this is linked with being overweight.

As I have mentioned before, this type of diabetes usually appears in people over the age of 40, hence its other name of 'adult-onset' diabetes. But there is a genetic factor too. Amongst South Asian and African-Caribbean people, for instance, the condition often appears after the age of 25.

However, recently, more and more children are being diagnosed with the condition, some as young as seven. Type 2 diabetes accounts for between 85 and 95 per cent of all people with diabetes.

So, poor diet, an over dependence on certain foods and a general lack of exercise are all great ways to give yourself Type 2. Which is how I ended up with it. I was guilty of all three.

Perhaps at this point I should tell you a little about myself – and my road to getting diabetes. When I was a kid I was skinny. Really skinny. Six foot tall and nine stone skinny. And no, it wasn't because I was a long distance running star. In fact when we had cross-country at school, the course very conveniently used to go past my gran's house. So I'd sneak into there on the way out and wait for all the bedraggled runners to come past again and join in at the end.

Even in my late 20s I still struggled to get past nine stone. I ate what I wanted and drank what I wanted. No problem. It might have been the cigarettes which kept my weight down, even if they did make me cough a bit sometimes. Then I hit the 30 mark and, without me realising it, my body's metabolism changed. Giving up the smoking at this time didn't help either – as I started to enjoy my food more because they tasted better! Suddenly I was buying new suits and shirts to fit my 12 stone frame.

Again, no problem. 12 stone is a good weight for a guy my height. But in 2002, I found myself in a job that was hugely stressful. I've always been in events and marketing and – believe me – it's a profession where stress is normal. Clients always want things yesterday. If something can go wrong, it will do. But in 2002 I found myself really up against it at work. I was working long hours and eating late. Being too late to go home and cook a meal, we would call into our local Indian, Chinese or Italian restaurant on the way home – whichever was still serving!

Although the food was fantastic – especially my favourite curries Lamb Balti or a King Prawn Dopiaza complete with a couple of naan breads and pappadoms. Bliss! But it was the wrong type of food at the wrong time.

And bliss, I found, was to come at a price. A heavy price! Without hardly realising it, I had ballooned out to 14 stone. And by 2004, when I was first diagnosed with diabetes, I was a couple of pounds shy of 15 stone and now starting to slow down noticeably.

I didn't hurry anywhere, and the only exercise I was getting was walking between my car and my desk. So I wasn't burning off the calories I was taking on board – they were just loading up my system and piling up the problems. And it was that deadly combination of poor diet, lack of exercise and working under extreme pressure that led to my bloodstream carrying a deadly load of unused fat and my body failing to properly cope with the glucose in my system.

So exactly what is going on in your body when you develop Type 2 diabetes? Here is the way it was explained to me.

Some scientific stuff!

The condition is also known as 'Diabetes Mellitus' – and there's a good reason for that. Diabetes, in Latin, means to 'siphon', or pass through. And 'Mellitus' means 'honeyed' or 'sweet'. So the urine of someone with this condition is literally sweet: it contains glucose that the body hasn't been able to process and use.

I found out one very interesting fact about diabetes: many years ago, before they had developed ways to accurately measure the amount of glucose in a person's urine, they would pour some near an anthill! If the ants came along, it showed that there was a lot of sugar in it. Thankfully, science has advanced somewhat since then.

Glucose is important stuff. It's the fuel that powers our body. When we eat or drink a carbohydrate, the gut converts that into glucose and releases it into our bloodstream. But to enable glucose to come out of our bloodstream and enter the cells of our body, it requires insulin – which is produced by the pancreas.

The insulin molecules effectively act as a key to unlock the cell – attaching themselves to the glucose molecules and allowing the glucose in.

In a healthy person, there's enough insulin to do this job, but in someone suffering from the more serious Type 1 diabetes, the insulin-producing cells in the pancreas have been disabled – so there's no 'key' to open the 'lock', and glucose cannot enter the cells. So it remains in the bloodstream – where excess levels can cause damage to the blood vessel walls, while the person starts to suffer from a dangerous lack of glucose in their body.

Type 2 diabetes is not so severe as this, but the complications can still be dangerous. In the majority of cases, the pancreas carries on producing insulin – but not enough for the body's needs.

And to add to the problem, the cells themselves build up a resistance to insulin – which is why it is known as 'insulin resistance'. The impact on the sufferer is that while their cells are being starved of glucose (which is why a common symptom is tiredness) the levels of glucose in their blood stream become dangerously high.

The effects of all that excess glucose coursing through your veins can be very harmful to blood vessels, which is why a common side effect of diabetes is damage to the eye and to vein walls. Blurred vision is a common symptom. The high blood sugar associated with diabetes actually make the lens of the eye swell, and is the leading cause of blindness in adults.

With nowhere else to go, some of the excess glucose in your system is flushed out through the urine – which is why there are typically high levels in the urine of a diabetic and why the person will be constantly thirsty: the body is losing liquid faster than you are taking it on board.

Your parents (and your parents' parents!) can also have a big say in whether or not you succumb to diabetes, because if two people had identical diets and lifestyles, there's no guarantee that both would develop diabetes. To some extent our genetics will determine how susceptible we are – which is why doctors will ask about your family history, and why certain races are more vulnerable than others.

Just getting older is also a factor for many people: about 20% of elderly patients in North America have diabetes.

Diabetes in the States is now a very serious problem – with 800,000 new cases being diagnosed each year. In the UK we've found ourselves being just behind the States on all sorts of health issues, notably obesity, so all the indications are that diabetes in the UK will get much worse in the coming years as the years of bad diet catch up on people.

Not everyone who has a bad diet, or is overweight, will get diabetes, but it is a big factor in Type 2 diabetes, and some 55% of those diagnosed with the disease are clinically obese. And there's another reason in addition to all the extra glucose in their bodies.

'Central obesity' (which is defined as the fat concentrated around the waist around our abdominal organs, but not subcutaneous fat) will actually predispose many people to insulin resistance. Why? Apparently, abdominal fat secretes a group of hormones called 'adipokines' which are believed to impair glucose tolerance.

The experts say that you are particularly at risk if your waist is 31.5 inches or over for women; 35 inches or over for Asian men and 37 inches or over for white and black men. And, of course, if you have a history of high blood pressure and strokes, the risk is significantly higher again. There are a number of other medical conditions which will predispose you, together with severe mental health problems.

How do you know if you have diabetes?

The problem, as I found, is that it's not always very obvious. Symptoms of type 2 diabetes may include:

- A constant and excessive need to urinate
- Constant thirstiness
- Tiredness
- Itchiness, especially in the genital area, and recurrences of thrush
- Sudden weight change
- Blurring of the vision
- Cuts and wounds not healing quickly

If any of these symptoms sound familiar to you, don't wait for a health check, as I did. Make an appointment with your doctor straight away! But all too often, we tend to ignore symptoms like this, or put them down to other conditions.

What is also worrying is that a great many of us have what is known as 'pre-diabetes' – our bodies are moving towards having full blown diabetes but have yet to exhibit all the symptoms. Even your blood sugar levels can be elevated, but aren't high enough to automatically mean a diagnosis. But anyone who has a health check and comes out with elevated readings should take this as a 'warning shot across the bows'.

And that is particularly the case if you are overweight, eating to excess or badly, not taking regular exercise or have a family history of diabetes. Each of these can be a contributory factor, and the more 'boxes' you tick, the more care you need to take! There is a very handy section on the Diabetes UK website that allows you to feed in information, and then assesses your risk factors. Try it!

It's also worth highlighting the importance of (at the very least) reducing and (ideally) stopping smoking. We all know the dangers of smoking, and how it can radically reduce your life expectancy. And I'm speaking as a reformed smoker myself. But if you have diabetes and you continue to smoke, it's a double whammy, because your body already has weaknesses which smoking will make worse. You will, statistically, significantly increase your chances of developing cardiovascular disease (heart attack, stroke or circulatory problems).

According to one study, 95% of diabetes-related amputations are carried out on smokers. Not great odds!

But don't take my word for it. Here I'm going to quote directly from the experts at Diabetes UK:

Smoking...

- ... when you have diabetes can make it more likely that you will develop neuropathy (nerve damage), nephropathy (kidney damage) and retinopathy (eye damage).

- ... decreases the amount of oxygen reaching the tissues of the body, which can lead to a heart attack or stroke.

- ... increases your LDL (low density or 'bad' lipids) cholesterol level and lowers HDL (high density or 'good' lipoproteins). This can make blood cells stick together, which can attract cholesterol and fats to stick to the artery walls making it more difficult for blood to circulate. This can damage and constrict the blood vessels of the body or cause a clot to form and possibly break away to travel round the body - leading to a heart attack or stroke.

- ... increases your blood pressure by releasing adrenaline which causes blood vessels to constrict and the heart to beat faster.

- ... raises blood glucose levels. This is probably due to the nicotine and other products involved in smoking which may cause insulin resistance (whereby insulin doesn't work properly) and stimulate stress hormones that can increase glucose levels.

In this book I talk mostly about how diet and exercise will give your body the chance to fight back against diabetes. But if you are serious – really serious – about getting better, you are going to have to stop smoking.

Lecture over!

So how can you treat Type 2 diabetes?

This is going to depend on how quickly you can have your condition diagnosed – and how much damage has already been done to your body's ability to produce (and make use of) insulin. Around 40% of Type 2 patients require insulin injections but for most people (60%) the medics will usually put you on a healthier diet together with an exercise regime – designed to get your weight down and reduce the potentially damaging amounts of glucose and fat in your bloodstream.

Fortunately, I fell into the latter category. I didn't need injections. But as every source of medical opinion will tell you, the best you can hope for is for the condition to ameliorate. But what I achieved was one better than that: I reversed the condition.

How? Read on!

Chapter 3
My first steps to reversing diabetes

"After the lecture that I got from the doctor, I was eating more carefully and I even started going to the health club, where I did a regular mix of half an hour in the gym followed by 10 or 12 lengths of the pool".

It would be great to tell you that I went straight from the doctor's, took my medication, ate a few salads and did a few runs round the block, and my diabetes sorted itself out. But of course it doesn't work quite like that. As you may have already realised from the date when I was first diagnosed, in 2004, it took me almost five years before I hit upon a way to get my body back under my control.

Along the way, I tried a few diets and even managed to shed two stone on several occasions. As someone once remarked about giving up smoking: "It's easy – I've done it dozens of times". So while the weight did come off, it wasn't long before my old habits began to creep up on me again. I ended up having a set of suits and shirts in my wardrobe, all of different sizes.

The problem was this: I found the diets I went on always left me hungry and short of energy. And while I cut back on my lager intake, the wine I had started to drink as a substitute was doing me no good either!

I once tried the 'Lipotrim' diet, which involved drinking milkshakes and lots of water. I certainly lost weight but after two weeks I felt really poorly, not helped by the fact that I really don't enjoy drinking water. I also had chronic constipation.

Yes, after the lecture that I got from the doctor, I was eating more carefully and I even started going to the health club, where I did a regular mix of half an hour in the gym followed by 10 or 12 lengths of the pool. But I was still under pressure at work – and finding it difficult to let the glasses of red wine go. So while I was more toned up... my weight was still bouncing around the 15 stone, or 210 pound mark.

Not good, even though my blood counts on cholesterol, triglycerides and glucose were much closer to an acceptable level – helped, of course, by a continuing regime of medications.

Then, shortly afterwards, I was introduced by a friend of mine called Giles to a diet that proved to be the best one I had found to date: the 'South Beach Diet'. He told me that it sounded ideal for someone like myself who was trying to battle overweight and diabetes. I bought the book, which is written by Dr Arthur Agatston, and agreed. This sounded more like it.

The book explains that as long as you eat the right carbs and the right fats, rather than the 'bad' ones, your body will start to shed excess weight. It allows you three healthy-sized meals a day plus a couple of snacks. This sounded like my sort of diet, and I not only began the diet – but also started looking into the science behind the book.

The book gives case studies of a number of people who have weight issues, several of whom have diabetes. They all share similar problems – but the situation for the patients with diabetes is more extreme. They would get hungry, and eat carbohydrate-rich food - and pump glucose into their body... not all of which could be absorbed because their insulin supply was inadequate.

Their bodies' natural reaction when that supply of glucose was no longer readily available, would be to crave yet more carbohydrates – even more so than those people who were just overweight without the added complications of diabetes.

The problem is that there are different sorts of carbohydrates. As I said earlier in the book, carbs aren't not just potatoes, rice and corn. A huge proportion of the food we eat contains carbohydrates in one form or another. From a glass of milk through to a piece of fruit, not forgetting alcohol, all of them contain sugar in a variety of different forms – and some release it as glucose into our bloodstream more slowly than others. The faster the release, the more of a 'sugar rush' we get.

In the last few years we've all got used to hearing about 'GI Levels' – the Glycemic Index that shows you which foods release their energy slowly and which do so more quickly. The whole concept was developed around 30 years ago from research by a Dr David Jenkins and others at the University of Toronto; tellingly, that research was designed to find out the best foods for diabetics.

In essence, those carbohydrates that break down quickly during digestion, and release glucose rapidly into the bloodstream, have a 'high GI', while those that break down more slowly, and release glucose more gradually, have a 'low GI'. Received medical opinion is that – for most of us, and particularly those with weight issues – on balance those foods with a low GI are more beneficial.

Look at the list and you can see why some foods give you a quick hit – but leave you feeling hungry – and others stay around and keep you feeling full for longer. The GI of multi-grain bread, for instance, is 48. A baguette is 95. Porridge is 49, cornflakes are 83.

According to the classification, low GI foods (those with a GI of 55 or less) will include most fruit and vegetables (except potatoes and watermelon), pasta, pulses (with the notable exception of broad beans), meats, milk, fish, eggs, nuts, cooking oil and brown rice.

Move up a category to medium GI foods (those with a GI of between 56 and 69) and you are talking about whole wheat products, most white rice and table sugar (yes, that surprised me too!).

The high GI foods include cereals such as corn flakes and rice krispies, baked potatoes, parsnips and (sadly) white bread... as well as most alcoholic drinks. Even fruits like dates (103) and watermelon (72) make that list.

It puts into perspective the idea that to be really healthy you can eat all the fruit and vegetables you want. For most of us, that's probably true (within reason!). But some fruits, most dried fruits and the majority of root vegetables are either medium or high GI foods. OK if your body is processing the glucose they generate correctly... not so good if it's not.

But even for those people without diabetes and simply

looking to shift a few pounds, it pays dividends to check out which foods will give them slow release energy (and so make them feel fuller for longer) and which might hit the spot quickly – but leave you feeling empty soon afterwards.

One quick guide if you are shopping in the supermarket and don't have a GI list with you, is that root vegetables are surprisingly high – they don't feature in my recommended list, that's for sure! Most other vegetables are less than 15 on the index – which is why they do!

One good piece of news for chocoholics amongst you is that your favourite treat is not as bad as you might think on the GI ratings – under 50. Which is why I've included it in my diet... albeit in modest amounts. If you have access to the web, you can find authoritative lists of the GI values of all the most common ingredients and processed foods – one good source - can readily be found on the Internet.

When a relatively healthy person eats a high GI food, the body responds to this quick release of sugar by releasing more insulin – and the blood sugar level then drops off again. Ironically, you can then get left with a craving for more sugar (it's called 'reactive hypoglycemia) and that is why 'slow release' carbs are better for you.

Just ask a marathon runner what they eat before a race and you'll find it's pasta the night before and porridge in the morning. Both give a steady release of energy into the body. They might top up with some jelly babies or an energy drink on the way round, but that's all it is: a quick-release top up to compensate for the huge amount of fuel they are burning.

But for a diabetic sat in front of a computer screen, the very last thing you want is quantities of glucose rushing round your bloodstream and which can't enter your cells – because your pancreas isn't producing enough insulin. It's a double whammy. More and more glucose builds up – you don't get the energy you need and long-term damage is being done.

And there's more. When the pancreas starts to falter, it stops doing its job, which is to produce insulin to process the fats that we eat – taking them to the cells in our body where they are used for energy, or stored in the form of 'triglycerides'. And that makes it doubly important that we eat the right fats too!

So olive oil features regularly in the menus that I started to develop, as do tomatoes and garlic – remember how the Mediterranean diet is meant to be one of the healthiest in the world. Interestingly, the addition of oil to a carbohydrate (for example, olive oil poured onto your pizza or pasta) will actually slow the digestion process down and render that carbohydrate 'slower'.

So it not only tastes better, but it's better for you too. And if you do what I do, and add some garlic into the oil, that makes it even healthier, as garlic is one of nature's natural healers. It has been used by centuries for fighting off infections and is now believed to help reduce cholesterol in the bloodstream.

You won't be totally surprised to hear that one omission from the diet – for at least the first few weeks anyway - is fruit. The fructose in fruit is a 'fast acting sugar' – and so gives you that quick lift, but then fades away, and most fruits (with a couple of notable exceptions) are in the medium GI band. So while it makes a reappearance later, for the first few weeks at least, no fruit! And no root vegetables either – especially beetroot, turnips, parsnips, potatoes and sweet potatoes. They too have high GI levels.

But there are plenty of low GI vegetables in there, so you will get your 'five a day' – and in larger amounts than you might expect!

And for any lager or beer drinkers out there, sorry, but that too has to go – certainly until you start to see your weight drop. The 'maltose' in beer has a phenomenally high GI level. Look at any regular drinker and see where they carry their spare weight.

Taking it one stage further...

As I mentioned earlier, the diets I tried in the first couple of years certainly helped shift the weight – each time by a couple of stones. And each time the weight reappeared. And the same was true of the South Beach diet. Not, I hasten to add, because it isn't an excellent diet. It really is. It's just that it didn't work for me long term. Adapting the diet to my tastes and adding in some other components that did work for me, was the turning point.

And that is what happened next.

In January 2009 I found myself working in Abu Dhabi for several weeks on a project. One evening I was sat with a friend of mine. We talked that evening about having control of our own lives and 'making it happen'.

It might sound clichéd, but somehow that was the resolve I needed. The way things had been going, the best I could ever hope for was to keep my symptoms under control. And still I'd be unhealthily overweight. At 45, that's not a good place to be.

But all my life, especially in business, I had prided myself on 'making things happen'. Taking responsibility for achieving my ambitions and not relying on others. Taking the inevitable setbacks on the chin and redoubling my efforts. Why should this be any different? No more excuses, my future was in my own hands.

I decided that I was really going to focus. It was time for a change.

We all get these moments in life. Crossroads, where we can choose to go in one of several directions. This was mine.

Of all the diets I had been on, the South Beach one had worked the best, and I had felt better on it. But still it hadn't kept the weight off. So that was the basis on which I developed MY version of a diet. Based on solid medical advice, but I also added in my own likes and dislikes – what I felt would work for me.

I also decided to ramp up my exercise regime from the fairly gentle (and not always regular!) sessions in the gym and the pool. More on that later!

Part of what made the new approach work for me was a shift in the way I looked at my diet. The battleground might still be my body, but I decided that my mind needed to control what was going on. I now looked upon the carbs in a simplistic way to make me feel more positively and negatively than I had before. Instead of 'good and bad' carbs, depending upon their GI index, they became 'nice and nasty'.

I told myself that they were either on my side – or against me. Helping to fuel my body... or clogging up my bloodstream.

I also knew, from the research that I had done, what to expect when I cut back on my intake and the 'carb cravings' started. Stop eating or drinking a food or drink you are used to consuming and your body will send out messages. "We want the same sort of food we've always had," they shout (or words to that effect!).

My approach? To look upon these messages as not coming from me – but from the chemicals in my body that were hooked on a certain sort of carb.

After all, who was in charge of my body: me or them?

And so when I gave up the foods I had been 'relying on', I told myself that it wasn't me that wanted them – but the chemicals in my body. It wasn't me going without, but them. I wasn't missing out on the treats and comfort foods I have enjoyed – they were.

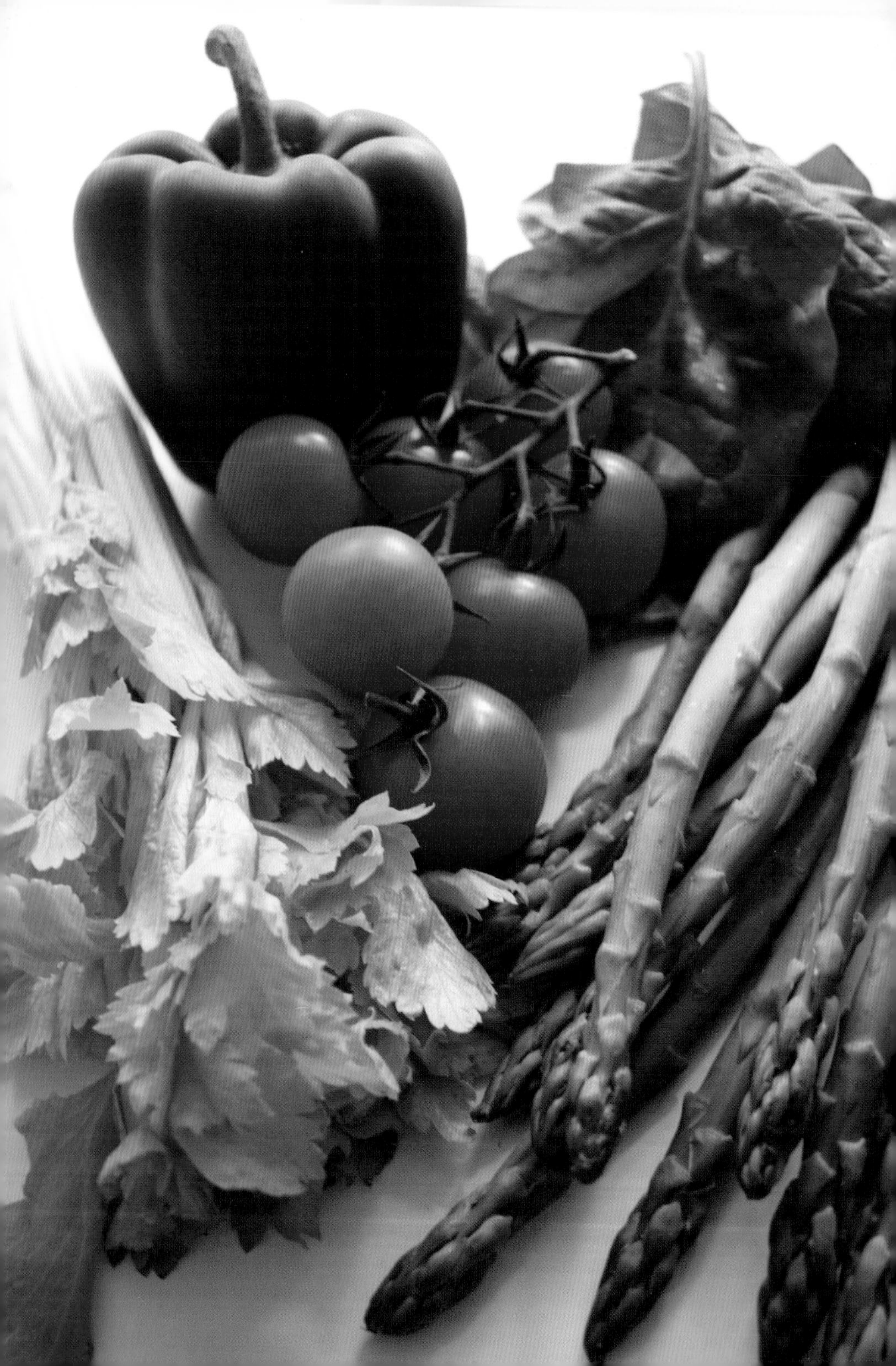

Chapter 4
I start the diet...

"So what were my 'famous five' ingredients? These are the ones that worked for me: celery, asparagus, spinach and green peppers were the four green fingers and tomatoes (which detox the body) was the fifth red thumb".

Photo - The key ingredients to my diet

In the early part of 2009, I set about adapting the diet that I had been on to my tastes. It was a good time to start. I had gone back up to 15 stone – the only way from here was down! I cleared out the cupboard of all the foods that I knew couldn't be with me on the first part of this journey and prepared a whole set of recipes and day-to-day menus that I felt would work best for me... again based on the science that I had read up on.

Most importantly, I only included foods that I knew I would enjoy eating. If I was going to be eating less food, it was critical that I make it things I would look forward to and regard as a treat... not a punishment.

I settled upon having five meals a day – three main ones and two snacks, because that would give me something to look forward to, and never more than a few hours away! I knew that my willpower would be stretched if I had to wait for four or five hours between eating.

I also wanted to make my life as simple as possible. I do have a busy existence, and so does my wife. We don't have the luxury of having a few hours each day to search out ingredients and create a constantly varying diet. I took the list of foods that I knew would fill me up – and release the energy I needed slowly - and simplified it to just five foods - four 'green' foods and one 'red' one – that I would build into my daily diet, and which would effectively take the place of the 'bad carbs' I was going to cut back on.

They would still give me energy, but more slowly.

I called the four green ones 'fingers' and the red one a 'thumb' – my simplistic way of remembering what I was eating.

All of them provide glucose in some form, but their GI level was as low as it is possible to be – under 15. These would release energy, yes, but very slowly.

In fact, several (notably celery) are regarded as being 'calorie negative' – they use up calories in the digestion process – while filling you up... how good is that? Effectively, they are 'sugar eaters'.

So what were my 'famous five' ingredients? These are the ones that worked for me: celery, asparagus, spinach and green peppers were the four 'green fingers' and tomatoes (which detox the body) was the fifth red 'thumb'. If you look at the list of other green and red foods, you'll find other options which you may prefer, but concentrating on having these in each day's meal simplified the whole process for me. I didn't have to keep thinking 'what shall I buy / cook / eat today?'

It was straightforward, simple even, and remarkably effective.

Having decided how I was going to go about my diet, I also resolved to make sure my body had plenty to think about in terms of exercise. As I mentioned a few pages back, I had started to go the gym – albeit not in a rigorous way. I would spend ten minutes or so on the cross trainer, push a few weights and then top it off by swimming a couple of lengths in the pool. Good – but not good enough!

I decided that I was going to step up my exercise routine alongside taking this new diet seriously. I'd tried dieting. I'd tried exercise. Now I was going to put the two together and make them work. All the reading I'd done had convinced me that through exercise I could increase my metabolism – and really speed up my weight loss. I wanted to do it inside a year – six months if possible.

An impossible ask? Not at all!

I got all my ingredients together and planned out my first day's meals – and this was how it went.

First off, breakfast. A good breakfast at that. Every good diet book will tell you not to skip the first meal of the day, and I had no intention of going to work hungry. I knew that if I did that I'd be stopping off and buying an energy bar, or snaffling a biscuit, and undoing all the benefits. My breakfast comprised asparagus and spinach omelette – with mushrooms added in for a treat.

I chopped the vegetables into bite-sized pieces and put them into the frying pan, together with some extra virgin olive oil, to heat them through and soften them up. As they were cooking, I whisked up two eggs and then tipped them into the pan. After a minute or two, I added a big handful of spinach on top of the omelette. After a short while, almost as it was cooked, I turned the omelette over and reduced down the spinach.
Absolutely delicious!

That was washed down with a cup of decaf tea – with skimmed milk, but definitely no sugar. I'm not a coffee drinker, but that could easily replace the tea.

That got me through to my mid-morning snack, by which time I was ready for a tasty morsel. The South Beach book recommends 'Laughing Cow' cheese triangles, and I found them very filling – and they are high on protein too. One 'Extra Light' triangle has just 19 calories – and it is over 50% protein. To go with it? Celery. Go on the Internet and you will see plenty of discussion about how digesting celery burns up more calories than it provides. No, I'm not sure how that works either: you'd think that might give you licence to eat whatever you want... as long as you ate copious amounts of celery!

But all I know is that it is filling, nutritious, with plenty of fibre – and a great snack when filled with a cheese triangle or two.

For lunch I wanted something that represented a treat that I could look forward to. So the night before I prepared a breast of chicken, which I had grilled to take out as much of the excess fat as possible. I took this to work with a lunchbox full of other delicious ingredients: more chopped up celery, spinach leaves, lots of plum cherry tomatoes (which taste incredibly sweet) and some green peppers (chopped). The whole meal was liberally drizzled with a mix of olive oil and balsamic vinegar with crushed garlic and chopped coriander.

Again, really delicious – and filling. And there was even a pudding: a Hartley's low sugar jelly. I was intent on keeping my 'sweet' tastebuds happy while I cut back on my carb intake.

During the middle of the afternoon, more protein: this time it was several slices of plain ham (although turkey would also do, both being lean meats).

Always my favourite meal of the day has been dinner, and the first dinner I prepared under the new regime set the trend. I also ate it early enough in the evening to digest it before I went to bed; a lot of health and diet books will tell you not to eat too late, as your body does not use up all the calories you consume – and then they are laid down as fat. One of the changes I made to my life was to shift the time I ate every evening to no later than 8.30, and this also made sure that I didn't fall into the temptation of dropping into my favourite curry house.

At the heart of the first meal on my new diet was a good slice of salmon or white fish, which I steamed to keep in all the goodness. Then, as a superb substitute for the potatoes I would normally have had (with a GI of 70), I steamed and then mashed half a cauliflower (less than 15 on the index) together with some Benecol spread, which has the added benefit of actively reducing your cholesterol.

Then pudding – yes, the second one of the day! I had half a 250g tub of ricotta cheese – Asda / Walmart's own make happens to be my favourite of all the brands I have tried –

topped with a teaspoonful of cocoa powder, half a teaspoonful of vanilla essence, a teaspoonful of fruit sugar (from Tate & Lyle) and a small handful of chopped chocolate chips.

All of that satisfied my sweet tooth – and I'm sure it will do the same for you.

That was my first day's meals and, I promise you, I went to bed without any hunger pains at all. I missed my evening drink, admittedly, but those would be totally empty calories that I really didn't need.

The recipes in the last section of the book set out lots more options – so you won't have to find yourself eating the same food day after day.

What's more, after a month you can loosen the diet a little and reintroduce a couple of constituents you will have missed.

Four greens...
Asparagus
Celery
Green pepper
Spinach

and one red
Tomatoes

This was the strategy to my diet - starting with the basics then introducing treats each month.

Month one

Strictly sticking to the main ingredients shown in my weekly diet plan on pages 118 to 124 with absolutely no alcohol.

Month two - five

Stick to the same diet plan but introduce some treats such as strawberries, bananas and low fat yoghurts. One glass of wine or a vodka & cranberry on a Friday.

Month six

Now I started to add some sauces to fish & meat meals, such as hollandaise and pepper sauces.

The rest of my life

Keep sticking to the main ingredients that are shown my hand on the right and limiting myself with carbs such as bread, pastries and potatoes. Vodka & cranberry on Friday and Saturday evenings only!

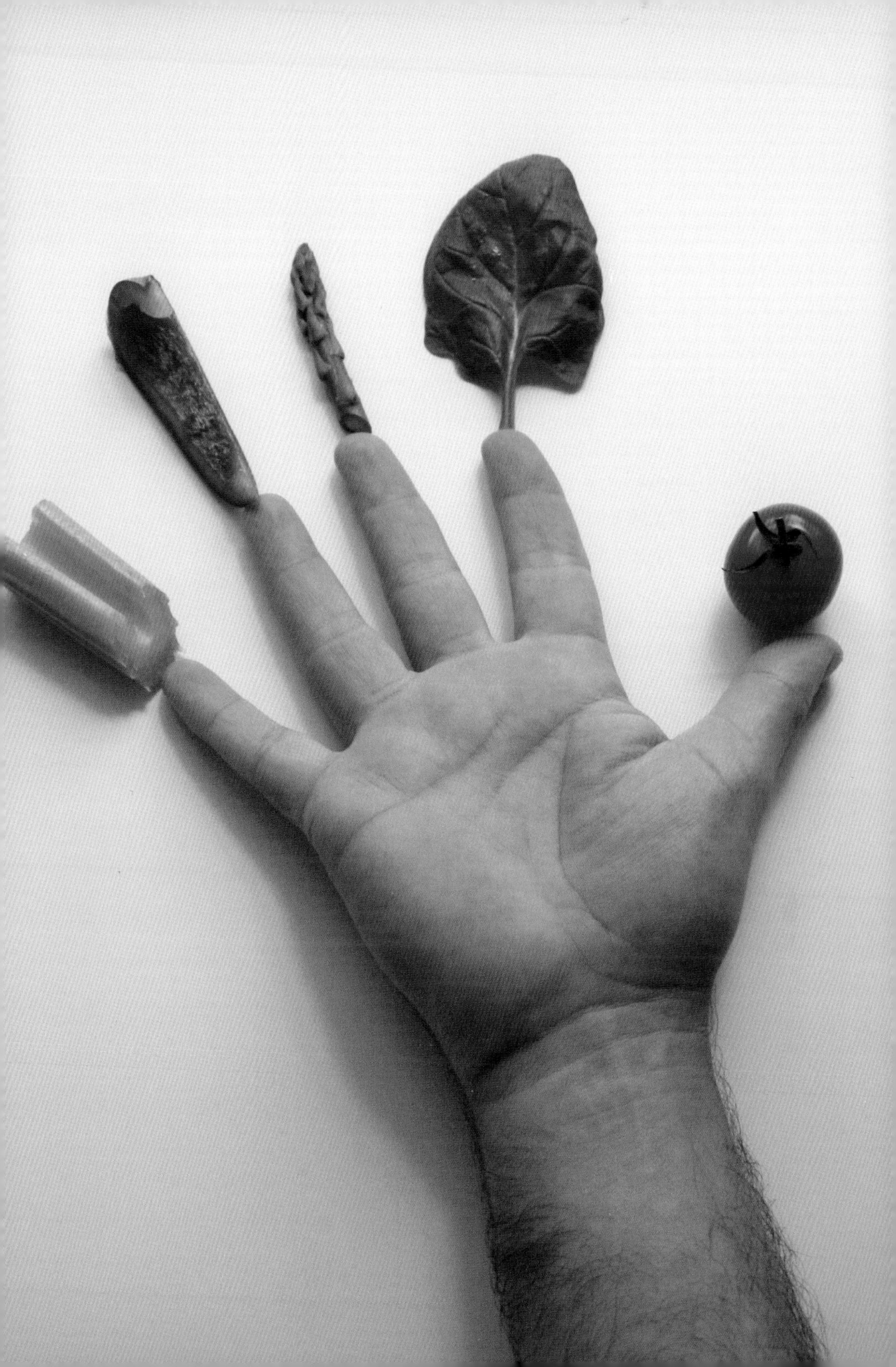

Watching the weight go...

Did it work? The first seven pounds that anyone loses during a diet are always the easiest. It pretty much comprises the excess fluid that the body carries around. So half a stone came off in just one week. By the end of the first month I was a whole stone lighter – so some real poundage was starting to shift. Most importantly, the second month was just as dramatic as the diet really kicked in and my exercise regime stepped up. Another stone went.

Month three and the weight loss was less dramatic – but still very steady: another seven pounds bit the dust. And it was the same in the next month – a further seven pounds reduction.

And if you think about it, it shouldn't be that hard. I was not taking on board calories that I couldn't burn and I was also, alongside that, increasing the amount I was burning up with exercise. I was getting my five a day fruit and vegetables – so no risk of hurting my health. And I was cutting back on the alcohol. I had none in the first month and then looked for the lowest offending drink I could. I started on vodka and slim-line tonic, never more than a double, and having cut out alcohol altogether for a while, that was enough!

However I then hit on a much better idea: vodka and cranberry juice. The vodka is not quite as bad as some alcohols, while the cranberry juice is a great 'detox drink' – so you're going some way towards compensating for what you're drinking.

Amusingly, a few months into my diet, when I was really showing a big difference in my waistline, I was in a hotel bar in Abu Dhabi with my friend. "So what's the big secret, Andrew?" he asked. "This," I joked, holding up my drink. "Vodka and cranberry juice."

It might have been said in jest, but before I knew it word had got around and everyone I met on my next visit seemed to have switched to Vodka and Cranberry...

As each month passed, I was able to relax the diet a little more. I added in bananas when I started running, and added orange juice after a while too – as well, of course, as the cranberry juice! I never did go back the beer and lager, though, but stick to a glass of wine or two at the weekend.

This level of abstinence might sound optimistic from where you are now, but curious things happen when you give up certain foods – especially the ones that give you a sugar rush. You find that you genuinely can wean yourself off them. Anybody who has given up sugar in their hot drinks will tell you that to drink it with sugar now takes sickly. It's the 'bad carbs' losing their power over you.

By the end of month four I had – incredibly - reached my initial target of 12 stone and was able to relax. But I was feeling so good, and really enjoying all the extra energy you have when you're not carrying extra weight, that I decided to keep on going down until my weight levelled off naturally. My natural weight turned out to be 11 stone – which is not surprising, looking at what I weighed as a young man.

Everyone, I think, has a natural weight – and that will depend on a huge number of factors. There is a big risk of people trying to go below that in order to be fashionable, and I'm sure that can't be good for you. But after six months I had lost four stone – and that was good enough for me.

If you look at a BMI table, that puts me at the low end of my 'ideal weight'. But to be honest I'm no Mr Universe – there was always a skinny person trying to get out of this body! However, that does allow me the luxury of a 'buffer' when I want to let my hair down from time to time – not that I have much hair to do that with! I have found on a number of occasions that if I go away on business for a week or so, particularly overseas, I'll come back four or five pounds heavier – mostly because it is harder on hotel and airline food to keep up your usual regime in that time. But that excess normally melts away fairly quickly.

In fact, because I was doing more running, which I'll describe later, I have been able to take some real liberties with my diet, reintroducing some of the carbohydrates that I had put to one side. But what was curious was that the yearnings for some of the 'bad carbs' that I had weaned myself off have never returned. Your body adjusts itself, and recognises what it really needs.

The beauty of this diet is that it is in phases: you don't start off on Day 1 thinking: "I've got to stay with this for months". It relaxes along the way – allowing you a few treats - and your body also adapts quickly so the cravings for certain foods recede. Yes, it takes some discipline, but it's the most enjoyable diet I have ever tried, as well as the most effective one.

By June of 2009, just six months after I began to seriously beat my diabetes, I had come down from 15 to 11 stone. More to the point, I went for a check up with my doctor and – effectively got a clean bill of health.

My cholesterol and triglyceride levels were healthy. My fasting glucose level was that of an average person too. I no longer take any medication. I can eat pretty much what I want – but having achieved a well and healthy body I would certainly not want to abuse it again, so 'all things in moderation'.

And something else remarkable had happened. One day I was in the sauna after a gentle work out and found myself getting dizzy. Rather than take a risk I went along to the doctor's who told me that my blood pressure was now too low – and that I had to come off the blood pressure tablets I had been on for over seven years. How good was that?

The medical profession may say that Type 2 diabetes cannot be 'cured'. Quite possibly if I decided to go back onto a bad diet and let my weight balloon again, the symptoms would reappear. But having none of the symptoms any more, I would go as far as to say that I have reversed it.

It's up to me now to make sure that it stays 'reversed'.

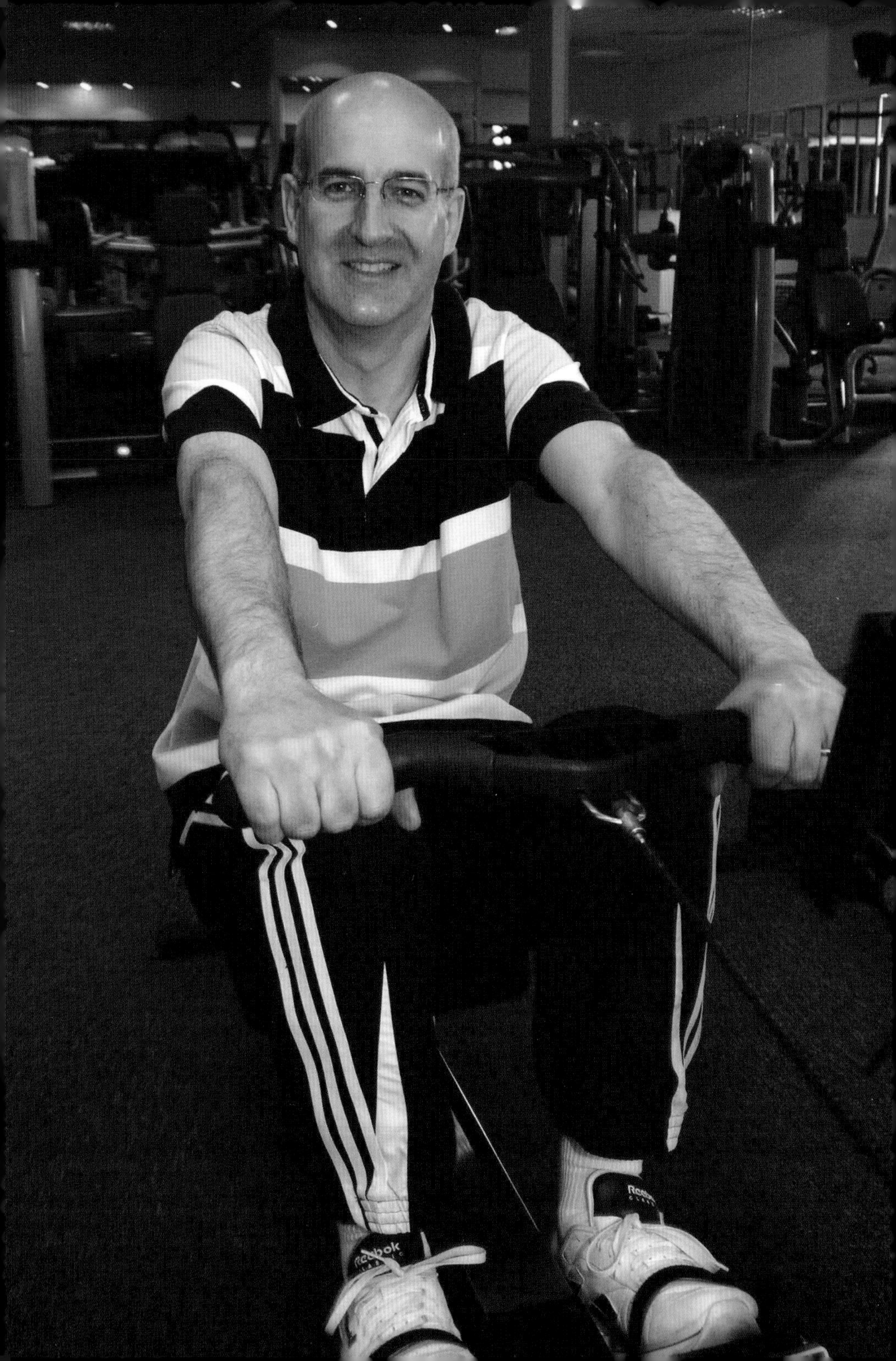
Reebok
Reebok

Chapter 5
Exercising

"Exercise was now my ally – it was on my side. Every time I got on an exercise bike, or started working the weights or machines, my body went further and further down the road to beating diabetes and being the shape and size I wanted it to be."

How do I put this? Exercise has never been my forte.

As I mentioned earlier on, I was always the kid at school who avoided exercise. So the prospect of some gentle exercise, as the doctor had recommended right at the beginning, was as off-putting to me as the thought of having to give up some of my favourite foods.

No matter how averse YOU are to exercise, believe me, I was there with you! So hopefully what I did to turn things around for myself will appeal to you – and at the very least demonstrate that it can be done.

As I mentioned, I did add exercise to my weekly timetable from when I was first diagnosed with diabetes. I can't say that I was very diligent about it – and that was one of the reasons I think my first diets never really stuck. Part of the process of 'taking control' of my body that I resolved to do early in 2009 was to make exercise a regular part of my life – and to 'reframe' it. By that I mean, not to look upon exercise (as it is so easy to do) as a chore... but as a vital means of helping me to win the battle I was fighting.

Exercise was now my ally – it was on my side. Every time I got on an exercise bike, or started working the weights or machines, my body went further and further down the road to beating diabetes and being the shape and size I wanted it to be.

The first thing that I realised was that my excuse for doing exercise, "I'm too tired", didn't wash. And that really helped.

In fact, what exercise does for you is to actually reduce the high glucose levels in your blood – so when you begin exercising you immediately feel less tired. Added to that, I was soon realising what people talked about with the 'endorphin rush' you get from exercise. It's very real, hugely enjoyable and, as many have discovered, somewhat addictive.

I have always focussed on exercising early in the morning – it suits me, as my energy levels then are at their highest. But other people seem to prefer doing something later in the day – in part because it fits in with their work schedule, but sometimes because they feel able to 'work out' their frustrations of the day on a bike, cross trainer or set of weights. It's whatever works for you! But do be careful about what and when you eat, and there is more advice on this later in the book. This is especially important for anyone whose diabetes is quite serious.

Scientists tell us that the body releases certain hormones into the bloodstream when you have exercised – partly to mask the discomfort you might well be in! But while that is true, there is another theory that part of that 'rush' you get after exercise, particularly if it has been hard work, is the 'high' you experience from overcoming a challenge.

I can certainly vouch for that. My own exercise pattern progressed through a series of stages. From doing a few hundreds yards on the treadmill right up to a half marathon. And from and not even a full length of the pool to confidently doing 20 lengths at a time.

I'm not saying you have to follow in those footsteps – everyone has to make a sensible plan depending upon their circumstances. Rush it, and the consequences can be quite serious - not only because your body well not be ready for too much exercise too soon, but also because of the particular problems and weaknesses that diabetes can cause.

But if you are living the life of a couch potato at the moment, look at it this way: not taking a moderate amount of exercise could seriously affect not only how long you live, but the quality of life you can expect. Surely that's worth breaking a few habits of a lifetime?

So what counts as exercise? Every form of exercise! To me, though, the key is finding something that you will enjoy, doesn't have to depend upon other people being there to help you, and doesn't cost the earth. Above all, it needs to be something that you can build up gradually.

Personally, my new fitness routine started off with some work in the gym on the cross-trainer and rowing machine, as well as some weights and swimming – a little of each to get the muscles working again, and nothing 'high impact' which would have put pressure on my joints.

But while most exercise is beneficial, a word of caution. Before 'setting off' on your new journey to fitness, do take medical advice. It's not just that you may be unfit (making it important not to put too much strain on your heart, joints and muscles too quickly too soon) but that having diabetes can damage your vascular system and nerves. That impacts

upon your circulation – and leads in turn to sore places not healing and becoming infected.
Your doctor or diabetes care team will make sure that you don't let your enthusiasm run away with you too quickly! So having had that check up, how hard should you push yourself? Gently does it, especially at first, is always the best advice.

Speaking personally, I'm a 'targets person'. I am motivated by thinking that 'I'm making progress'. I love to set myself a challenge and then meet it. It's not necessarily about being competitive, but about being the best you can be. If that sounds like you, then think about ways to keep yourself motivated: for instance, if you are able to walk, walking is brilliant as it not only gets the weight down but the blood circulating too. And getting a step counter is an excellent way of 'keeping yourself honest' – you can't pull the wool over a step counter's eyes because it doesn't have any!

You may have heard of the 'ten thousand steps a day' exercise. And it's a cracking idea. But if you are carrying too much weight, or you are suffering from some of the medical conditions that often accompany overweight and diabetes, 10,000 steps is a long-term goal – not something you can expect to do straight away. Start with one or two thousand steps a day (you'll be reassuringly surprised how few that actually is over a day!) and 'kick on' from there!

You can avoid making it a chore by building in lots of little walks into a day. Stop getting into the car for very short journeys. Get off the bus one stop early. Don't try and find the car parking space closest to the supermarket – find one a little further away. Use the stairs instead of the lift and, if a friend has a dog, why not invite yourself to go along one day – and then perhaps offer to walk them occasionally. A dog can never have too many walks!

Step counters can cost you anything from a fiver upwards, but obviously the more you pay the more sophisticated they are going to be. The better ones actually have built-in features which allow to you see your activity over a period – and so set yourself targets, and it will assess how many calories you have burned off (another great incentive!).

How many you burn will depend upon the speed you walk at, how hilly it is and how much you weight. But an average person of average weight uses up around 100 calories a mile.

What step counters will do is make EVERY short walk purposeful, even moving about the house or garden, and keep your mind on the positives of losing weight and tackling your diabetes.

Join your local gym or health club (as I did) and you'll have access to treadmills which can be set to ANY pace (from that of an arthritic snail upwards!), and to any gradient too. The scenery isn't necessarily riveting, granted, but in a gym you're immune to the weather and dark nights, and many of them have big screen TVs to while away the miles.

My fitness 'mission' started off on a cross trainer, before moving onto a treadmill, working up from something slightly above walking pace up to a jogging pace, before I took to the road.

Swimming

Walk for a long distance can be tough if you are carrying a large amount of weight, but swimming won't put any strain on your joints. Not all of us are confident swimmers, especially if we are self-conscious about our appearance, but there are classes that specialise in helping people get their fitness back; others provide non-swimmers the lessons and confidence they need to get going.

Frankly, you will be amazed at how quickly you will find that a first few lengths (or widths) of your local pool will soon build up. When I began I couldn't even manage a whole length of the pool – I was that unfit, and I also couldn't master the (rather necessary) art of swimming and breathing at the same time. But within a few months I was up to 20 lengths in a session. A half hour in the pool can burn up anything between 250 and 400 calories.

Swimming is, without doubt, one of THE great exercises for anyone trying to get back into fitness and wanting to shed unnecessary poundage, although not quite as quickly as running. Most towns and all cities have pools, and it's one exercise where you need very little investment in kit – although a costume is advisable! It has been one of my three principal forms of exercise in my regime – and has played a vital role in burning up calories, gently increasing my metabolism and improving my well-being.

Swimming will exercise your whole body – but without the risk of straining joints and muscles. You can use the stroke that's most comfortable for you and you will be absolutely amazed how quickly your endurance levels increase.

Of course it helps if you can swim! If you feel you need to gain more confidence in the water, every public pool runs adult lessons – both for beginners and those that are looking to sharpen their technique, and staff can sometimes take on the role of a personal trainer. How hard you push yourself is up to you, but it is always advisable to start gently before you try and perform any heroics.

Warming up and stretching before starting your swim is important to prevent injuries. For swimming, the most important stretches are the pectorals, the shoulder girdle, the calf muscles, the hamstring muscles and the quadriceps muscles. These can be done in the pool or before you get in.

Rowing

How many of us watched the phenomenal feats of Sir Steve Redgrave, Matthew Pinsent, James Cracknell and the rest of the Olympic heroes and thought "I'd like to do that?"

Well not that many, probably, as it did look like very, very hard work. All they could do after they won was to fall into each other's arms, narrowly averting a dunk in the water... and those competing in the annual boat race often DO end up in the River Thames.

Of course at that level it all looks incredibly hard work, which makes it even more important to point out that the greatest rower of them all, and our greatest ever Olympian, is Sir Steve Redgrave. And all those exhausting training sessions, as well as the races themselves, were undertaken with him suffering from diabetes. It certainly didn't seem to stop him: he learned to combine his passion for the sport with taking the necessary precautions of managing his condition, consuming up to 7,000 calories a day (no, that wasn't a misprint!) and having insulin injections.

In fact, rowing on a gym machine can use even more calories than swimming – obviously depending upon how much effort you put in. I don't recommend 7,000 calories a day's worth, unless you are a phenomenal athlete like Sir Steve, but it does allow you to burn up fat and justify having a more relaxed diet!

Rowing uses a whopping 70% of the body's muscles dynamically, so it burns a lot of calories. How many? A moderately fit person can burn between 600 and 1000 calories an hour. A very fit one over 1200. Even going fairly gently will use up between 350 and 500 an hour.

But the big benefits of rowing are that it doesn't put the same strain on your joints as walking, it works your whole body – upper as well as lower – improves your flexibility and really stimulates your cardiovascular system. Indoor rowing machines are the staple of every gym these days and, if you're serious, you can buy one too.

The indoor variety of the sport is claimed to be one of the fastest growing activities in the country, and some people take it very seriously indeed – with competitions and national and regional records being set. I'm not in that league, but what does provide an incentive to keep on going is that you can see just how far you have rowed.

I just loved being on the machine – and even a few minutes' each day worth will pay dividends. Every gym and health club will have several rowing machines and you don't have to be an Olympian to do it – and you can build up your endurance and speed at your own pace.

Weights and exercise machines

My early exercise routine also included sessions with free weights (those are the small and large dumb bells that you will find in any gym. I focussed on the smaller ones!). These aren't so important for losing weight, as they won't burn up calories in the same way as running, swimming, cycling or rowing will. But they do tone your body up. And if you find that underneath the first layer of flab is another layer of flab... you might want to tone up what you have got!

I built in twenty minutes doing these, three times a week, together with time spent on the other exercise machines – the cross trainer, and occasionally the rowing and cycling machines – which gave me a cardio-respiratory work out as well as building my stamina. I didn't go at it hell for leather, and always finished with some lengths in the pool and a few minutes' relax in the sauna. I found it an hour that I really looked forward to, not something I dreaded.

So that was my exercise routine. I'm not saying it's the right one for everybody – everyone has to go at their own pace – but it worked for me.

The end result was that I was starting to average burning up around 2,000 calories a week. Bear in mind that a pound of fat is some 3,500 calories, and you can see that – even if I didn't diet – I would be losing a couple of pounds each month. Equally, it was stimulating my metabolism, so that it got used to burning calories – and all the medical evidence points to exercise kick-starting our body's ability to combat insulin resistance.

More to the point, the exercise I was taking was balanced – using both my upper and lower body – and while never putting excessive strain on my cardio-respiratory system, it gave my heart and lungs a solid work out three times a week.

When I had lost enough weight, I added in running – first on the treadmill and later on the road. Fifteen stone is a lot of weight to take jogging, but 11 stone has proved easy. But more on that later!

The exercises I set for myself suited my interests and my circumstances. But there's no reason to restrict yourself to what I did. Cycling, dancing, horse riding, weights... all of them will help improve your fitness. But whatever you do, stick at it – and remember that different exercises and sports offer different advantages.

- Those that get you slightly out of breath and with an elevated heart rate are the 'aerobic' exercises that will work your cardiovascular and respiratory systems (your heart and lungs).

- Strength training – using weights especially – will build stronger bones and muscles.

- Flexibility training – such as pilates and stretching – are highly beneficial to diabetes sufferers because they keep your joints flexible, reducing the chance of injury and enabling you to move about more freely (and so encourage you to do more exercise).

A balance of all of these is helpful. But my principle aim with my exercise regime was the same as with my diet: look at it scientifically and logically and then develop one that suits you - one which you can actually enjoy. If you don't, you'll almost certainly end up as one of those people who have a cupboard full of barely-used exercise equipment... and still sporting an oversized tummy.

If these forms of exercise don't appeal...

... try cycling.

A recent survey found that those who 'get on their bikes' for at least 20 miles a week reduce their chances of heart problems by half. For anyone carrying too much weight, or suffering the circulatory problems associated with diabetes, that has to be very good news indeed.

Cycling burns up anything from 300 calories an hour too – more if you are pushing yourself – and it's the one exercise that (after your initial investment in a bike and helmet) could actually save you money!

I have to say that, as a former fattie, I also think it's a great sport for anyone carrying some extra avoirdupois: you can still bowl along (although hills will always provide a challenge) and not suffer from damage to your joints and ligaments. If you're anxious about cycling on our roads (or pavements as some cyclists seem keen on doing) there are many traffic-free routes where you can build up your skills and confidence.

Variety is the spice of life...

As I have made plain throughout, the diet was the key way in which I lost weight. But exercise has played a massive part in me regaining my health and well-being, as well as trimming the extra pounds.

Running, swimming and gym, with rowing thrown in for good measure, were crucial to improving my cardio respiratory system. They also helped tone up my body. So less fat was circulating in my system, surplus glucose was mopped up and my whole body's metabolism was speeded up.

There are many of us – too many – who are looking for quick fixes to losing weight and achieving the body of their imagination. My advice is that you will need a bit of willpower if you want to really reach your goals – and the exercise regime I went through was never taxing, but it was hugely rewarding.

The secret, I believe, is to mix it. I could never have been out in all weathers running – especially living in Wales. And neither would it have been a balanced exercise. Neither could I have limited myself to just sitting on a rowing machine, pumping weights or going up and down a pool. I have a very low threshold of boredom and so the perfect solution for me was to mix the activities.

The benefits have been enormous. I haven't suffered any injuries along the way, I haven't dropped out through tedium and my whole body is that much fitter – not just part of it. Because you are using different muscles and joints in different ways, you can actually exercise more. Every runner's magazine will tell you to 'cross train' for optimum fitness – and the same would be true of other sports too.

Finally: whatever exercise you take up, build up gently, warm up before you start, warm down after you finish, try a mix of exercise and – if you do get an injury – don't try and train through it. It can often turn a minor niggle into a longer-term problem. And if you think you need some medical assistance, get it!

My typical gym workout per week - 50 minutes per session

3 minutes rower
10 minutes cross-trainer
15 minutes weight machines
7 minutes bike
Total 35 Minutes

Followed by 15 minutes swimming

This was my main activity three times a week - Monday, Wednesday and Friday mornings before work.

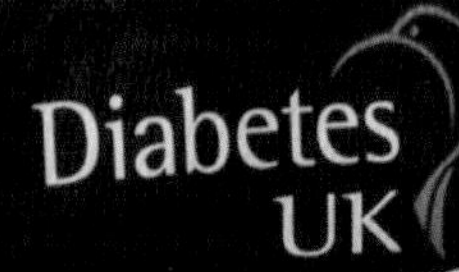
Diabetes
UK
CARDIFF HALF MARATHON 2009
5197
asics
www.diabetes.org.uk

Chapter 6
How running helped me

"To feel the breeze tugging at your cheeks, appreciate the beautiful countryside on either side, and the warm sun on your face... this was what I'd been avoiding all those years. What's more, I felt absolutely brilliant."

The diet that I have outlined in Chapter 4 played the biggest single part in me losing four stone in six months – and putting diabetes behind me. But the exercise regime definitely played a big part too – and probably tipped the balance. It increased my body's metabolism, helped give me more energy and burned off the excess glucose circulating in my system.

Every doctor or diabetes care team will tell you the same: exercise as much as you can – but very carefully!

Swimming, gym work and the rowing machine were really helpful parts of my exercise regime – but more on those later. The next few pages are designed to encourage you to start running. I never started off a runner, but now it's one of the most enjoyable and rewarding things I do – and I would like to share that with you.

I know, people who aren't natural runners are hardly good advertisements for the sport – puffing and perspiring along our pavements. But believe me, if you can get through the first few stages of discomfort (and embarrassment) there are few better ways to get in trim. Combined with cutting back on the wrong foods and eating the right ones, running will make a massive difference to your weight loss and wellbeing. Trust me on this. I was the world's most reluctant runner – now I can't wait to get out there. And this is how I did it.

My first step (literally) was onto a treadmill. Every gym and healthclub has one and they have one big advantage: you never get wet or cold on one. They're the perfect starting point as you can set your own (very modest) speed and distance targets and then set about achieving them.

I began at a quick walking pace (4mph / 6kph) which made me stride out at a faster pace than I would normally go. It was just a half mile the first time, then a stop to check my heart rate, and off for another half mile. And that was it. Just one mile in my first session. It wasn't really running, but I had pushed my heart rate up, got a warm glow going and – at the end – felt better for it. Most importantly, I hadn't overdone it on the first time out and injured or pulled something.

The next time I went, a couple of days later, I was eager to push the speed and distance up, but kept it to one mile at the same very modest fast walking pace, followed by a break, then another half a mile. And for the last four hundred yards I speeded the treadmill up to 7mph – a very modest jogging pace.

At that pace, there are no dangers – you can easily reach the 'stop' button if you feel uncomfortable and, if you are anxious, actually hold an emergency cord in your hand.

Go along to any gym and – as well as the annoying superfit looking types pumping weights – you'll see plenty of people just like I was, and possibly you are now. Doing just a mile or two at walking pace or not much above. So don't be too embarrassed to join their ranks – you have as much right to be there as the people going at 10 mph or pumping weights.

I know other people who may not have gym membership, or who want to establish a base level of fitness before they 'go public', and who start doing very short jogs during a walk – perhaps from one lamppost to the next – before taking a breather, walking for 30 or 40 yards. Then, with their breath back, they'll run another short stretch. Gradually you will find yourself walking less and running more – promise! – and it's an excellent way to start.

The next stages

Over the next few months I gradually (and I mean gradually) increased the distance and speed on my treadmill and started to add in more quicker sections to get my heartrate up. I even set the 'incline' to 1 and then 2 degrees – enough to make it more of a challenge and prepare me for the next stage of my journey – going out on the road.

When I was comfortable running three miles at 6mph – or 10-minute miling – I felt ready to put my new found fitness to the test. This was in June 2009. My weight had now come down to just 11 stone, so even if I wasn't running fast, at least I looked the part.

The first test was a short course starting at the entrance to the health club I go to. I wasn't alone. Alex from the Vale Hotel Golf & Spa Resort, Hensol, near Cardiff (where the Wales rugby team train) offered to come with me. He said it was for company, but I suspect it was to make sure that I didn't keel over because the Club would lose a member! The weather was perfect: a deliciously warm early summer's day.

The route was definitely not as flat as the treadmill – after all, this was Wales. At the end, I felt weary – it had definitely been tougher than running in the gym but infinitely more enjoyable. To feel the breeze tugging at your cheeks, appreciate the beautiful countryside on either side, and the warm sun on your face... this was what I'd been avoiding all those years.

What's more, nothing hurt, nothing had dropped off and I felt absolutely brilliant. I'd done it in just over 30 minutes – not electric, but respectable. More to the point I had no ill effects – in fact, my energy levels felt great. I was hooked.

Over the next few weeks I followed the advice of a running friend of mine: don't try to do too much too soon. I gradually extended the length of the run and soon found myself doing four miles with comfort, as well as two or three shorter sessions on the treadmill each week. I was still doing some gym work and swimming – and the combined effect was to enable me to take a few more liberties with my diet.

As fantastic as it was to reach my target weight, my wife Bev was quick to point out that there is such a thing as 'too slim'. I certainly found that if I had a couple of pounds 'spare' I didn't get the hunger pains between meals, or the feeling that I was about to run out of energy.

But as happy as I was with my running, something was niggling at me. I'd run further than I'd done in my whole life – the previous 'best' was from school to my gran's. How far could I go? My running friend, Tony, invited me over to go out with him – to check my progress by going out with him for a run. This was my chance to push the boat out – and see how far I could go.

"You can't go out looking like that," was the first, encouraging thing he said when he saw me kitted for the run. "What do you mean? Like what?" I demanded.

Perhaps I should mention at this juncture that my friend takes his running a bit seriously. He's 57, but runs about 30 miles a week and his best time in 2008 was 1.33 for a half marathon. That's seven minute miling – three minutes a mile faster than I was managing. So I felt obliged to listen to him politely at the very least.

"Look at your shoes," he said. "You've got to get some proper running shoes or you'll damage yourself. And new socks, proper running socks. And new shorts, proper running shorts that let you run freely."

"What's wrong with my shorts? I play tennis in them OK."

"And what's that top you're wearing?"

"It's an old polo shirt."

Tony was stood there like Mr Nike – with all the kit. He even had one of these wristwatch type 'Garmin' devices that has an inbuilt satellite connection, and tells you how far you've run, where you've run, how many feet you've climbed and even how many calories you've burned up. He had to know what he was talking about if he was wearing one of those. "Well," he said as long as you don't mind getting blisters, a chafed crutch and nipples, what you're wearing is just fine."

I hadn't realised running was quite so dangerous. But with nothing else with me to change into, we set off for our run – me very apprehensive, and Tony promising to stay back with me, whatever pace I went. "What's our target?" he asked. "Five miles," I said confidently.

"Let's go then."

I confess I was a bit worried. He lives in Cheddar – which has some very large hills, not least the Gorge itself. But fortunately we went to run around the local reservoir – a circular 2.2 mile route which couldn't be much flatter. "We'll go twice round," he said, "and then a bit more - I'll tell you when we hit the five mile mark."

We set off at a steady pace, our partners going in the opposite direction – so that every so often we would pass them and they could give us an encouraging wave. It was a perfect day for running. Warm but not hot, a gentle breeze blowing – and some fabulous countryside to make you forget the discomfort. Looking to one side we could see the Gorge – a huge ragged scar in the green Mendip Hills – and to the other, Glastonbury Tor was just visible. And as we headed in the opposite direction, there was South Wales glinting in the sunshine.

As I keep saying – running has some wonderful plus points!

Because he was wearing a Garmin, Tony kept telling me exactly how fast I was going, and I kept up a steady 9.30 minutes for the first mile – and the second. By the end of the first circuit, I was starting to slow a little – but still feeling good. We slowed to 10-minute miles for the second lap, and I now knew that I had really run further than I'd ever run before. But as we approached the five-mile mark, I made my mind up. I was not going to stop yet!

Instead we kept on running – and running. Past the six mile mark – and just over a half a mile to the end of the third circuit. I even managed a sprint finish at the end and, as we got there, my arms automatically went up in the air to the cheers of my wife and friends. I had done it! 6.6 miles.

I know it sounds insignificant to many people who can run marathons – and more. But just months before I'd been a physical mess – four stone overweight, struggling with diabetes and seriously unfit. I had run further than a 10k race – and 50% of the way to a half marathon.

I felt on top of the world – and didn't hold back when we had dinner that evening – I'd earned every mouthful!

Even Tony was astonished at what I had done. "Nothing's hurting?" "Well, yes – but not too bad." "Well if you can do that, you could do a half marathon inside three or four months if you put your mind to it."

Me? A half marathon? 13.1 miles? Well why not? As I have always maintained, what you can do is often limited by what you think you can do. And three months would give me a chance to run in my local half marathon, Cardiff. If I can run that far – why couldn't I run as far again? As Tony was quick to point out, there's a big difference between 6.6 miles and 13.1. If I was going to get round that course in reasonable shape – and without injuring myself – I was going to have to do it properly.

"And the first thing you do," said Tony, "is to get to a running shop!"

In fact it was the second thing I did – the first was to enter the Cardiff Half Marathon online. As soon as I saw my entry was accepted I sent out an email to all my friends: "What have I done?.. oh and here is my fund raising page on the web." If I was going to get over the finish line of a 13.1 mile race I was determined that Diabetes UK Cymru would get the benefit of that!

Some cautionary notes

As I have mentioned several times, if you are going to increase your physical activity and you have diabetes, you will need to take some sensible precautions.

When I started my fitness regime I took advice from my doctor – being in one's 40s, and having a history of diabetes, high cholesterol and blood pressure as I did, you do have to be careful! If your surgery has a diabetes team, they will be pleased to talk through your plans with you.

So what do you need to be aware of? Here is the best advice I can give – with assistance from Diabetes UK.

People with diabetes can be prone to foot and circulation problems. So you do need to ensure you are wearing appropriate footwear for your activity.

If you plan to take up running, your footwear is doubly important. I started off using my old pair of cross trainers. Bad idea. As soon as I stepped up my mileage my knees started to creak and my hips ached. Running puts huge stresses on your feet and ankles – the weight going onto them is far greater than your actual body weight, and that happens hundreds of times times every mile!

The first rule of running is not to start off too quickly – gently does it as you get your heart and lungs 'up to speed'. And don't 'up' your mileage too quickly either, however well you feel you are doing – a couple of miles a week extra is quite enough, otherwise your body will find it hard to adjust to the new stresses and strains you are putting on it.

The second is to invest in a proper pair of trainers. Which ones though? Looking at the array on offer is enough to make you dizzy. However if you go to a shop that specialises in running (every city and many larger towns will have one) they will put you on a treadmill and watch you run. They can then do a computerised 'gait analysis' which tells them what sort of shoe to recommend. And take in your old trainers when you go. Why? Because that will give them an important clue as to whether you 'overpronate' (strike the ground on one side more than the other).

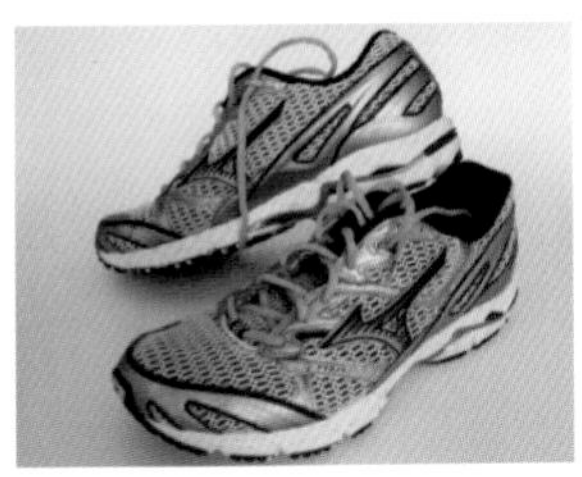

Don't expect to get much change from £70 or £80 for a pair which will not only protect your feet and legs, but also make you feel like a proper runner!

While you are in the shop, you will also need to buy some running socks. They are far better at absorbing the moisture when you run, so preventing rubbing and blisters.

The other 'no-no' of even semi-serious runners is the t-shirt. They're a convenient top to wear, but as you perspire, the moisture stays where it is – so at the end of a long run your top feels like a dead weight and you look like a wet rag. And yes, you can get chafed nipples, and they do hurt – especially when you get into the shower afterwards! A proper 'technical' running top will 'wick' the moisture away from your body keeping you a lot cooler as well as drier.

So shoes, socks, shorts and a top. This, I have discovered, is the basic 'kit' you will need if you are going to move off of the treadmill and onto the road / footpath.

If you start to take it more seriously, the next raft of useful items include a reflective top so that drivers can see you, especially if the light is poor, and a shower-proof top to wear in wet weather. Then there are the leggings that will keep you warm when it starts to get cold! Most of us who start to run get put off when the weather is poor – or the nights close in. With the right kit, you can keep running all year round – and keep the fitness you have fought so hard to attain.

Once you start to gain some confidence, you might want to check out if there is a running club nearby. Despite what you might think, most clubs have a very wide spread of ages and abilities and will usually welcome new members. Most are incredibly supportive and will give you advice on how to improve and avoid injuries.

My first race... and the 10 mile mark

My next big landmark was to run 10 miles. I'd been thinking of it for a few weeks and gradually increasing my long weekend run to eight miles. But first, I had the chance to take part in my very first race. Kidney Wales was organising a 10k race in Cardiff – the perfect opportunity to find out what it was like to run with several thousand other people.

It was a large field, with (as you'd expect) everyone from flyers to dawdlers taking part. One chap had tagged onto me near the beginning and told me that I was going to be his pacemaker. He dropped back after a couple of miles, which made me sorry for him – but also boosted my self confidence. It was hugely reassuring to find that – as slow as I was and only ever having run between 10 and 15 miles in a week – I could still beat a third of the field and came home in 57 minutes. I felt tired at the end of it, but buoyed up to think I had come this far, this quickly.

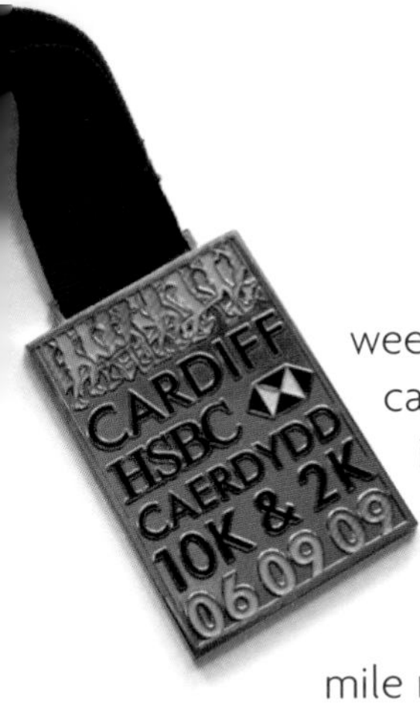

The first time I reached the psychological 'ten-mile mark' was on a trip to Nova Scotia. As part of my work as a marketing consultant I found myself in Halifax (no, not the West Yorkshire one!) and with a few hours on my hands. The scenery there is absolutely fabulous and, even if Halifax is the capital of Nova Scotia, it's still a small city by British standards (a bit bigger than Cardiff) and very clean and green. Also like Cardiff, it is a city whose fortunes have been made by it being a port, and my run took me from the centre down to the docks and back – overlooking the very picturesque bay on which the city stands.

At the end I was sore – but nowhere as bad as I had feared. The pace hadn't been electric... something over 9.30 miling... but for someone who had run so little, I was more than happy.

I never did get a 'Garmin' to tell me how far and how quickly I had run. Instead I discovered there is an 'app' for my iPhone which does a pretty similar job... and no need to splash out either. What's more, a very sultry lady's voice tells me each time I complete a mile - which is pretty neat. I had a huge sense of satisfaction from the ten mile run, and was buoyed up to know that, if I could run that far, just three more miles would take me to a half marathon.

That milestone came just a few weeks later, on October 18th 2009. It was barely three months since I had managed that breakthrough 6.6 mile run and, in truth, I really hadn't done the mileage my running friend had advised me would be the minimum to get round in comfort – and certainly not within the two hour target I had set myself.

But the day couldn't have gone better. The Cardiff Half Marathon is one of the flattest there is and, I'm assured, one of the best organised. I was lucky enough to be part of the Diabetes UK Cymru 'team' and so had my kit taken off me at the starting line – and kept for me until the end. It was a delightfully cool, sunny morning too with scarcely any breeze. Perfect!

I'd decided to try and keep at around nine minute miles for the first ten (if I could) and then see what was left. That way, if I WAS going to get a sub-two hour time, I would have a chance.

All the way through I felt fairly comfortable and was careful to stop at all the water stations. I found that I was just behind the nine-minute mile mark – but only just. Perhaps, I thought, if I could give it a push in the last three miles... But like so many before me, the ten mile mark – the furthest I had run, and never as quickly as this – was when the energy started to drain out of my legs. I found myself slowing slightly but I gritted my teeth and kept going, encouraged to see others around me starting to stop and walk.

Those last three miles were hard, hard work – but with the

end in sight I managed something of a sprint for the last 'point 1' of a mile and came in on 2 hours, 02 minutes. Not bad for a first timer!

I must say that three things kept me going over the last few miles. One was the promise of a Sunday roast when we got home. Second was the challenge I had set myself when I first managed to run over six miles. And third was the fact that I had sponsorship for Diabetes UK Cymru to the tune of over £500 riding on it. I was going to make that finishing line and collect my medal, hell or high water.

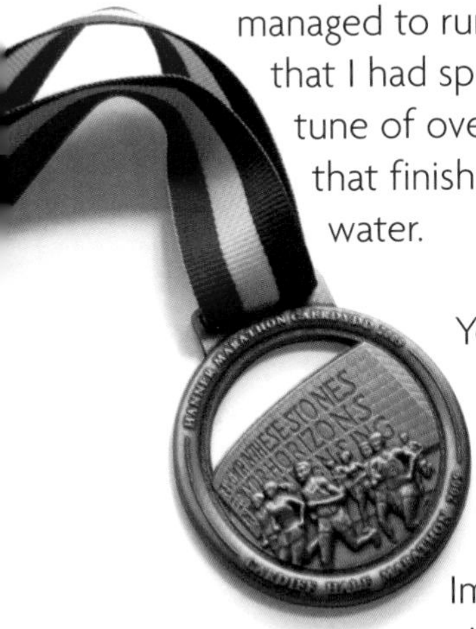

Yes, I was 5339th out of 11,000 entries - 8812 actually finished so 5661 people passed the finish line behind me. The other 2,188 entrants sadly didn't even make it.

Importantly, even after all that rigorous exercise, my body held up, with no signs of the hypoglycaemia that can affect diabetics if you 'run out of steam'. It's worth including a quotation here from the Diabetes UK website, that: "Regular exercise increases insulin sensitivity. Endurance athletes who treat their diabetes with insulin may sometimes reduce the amount of insulin they inject while training."

I, of course, was fortunate enough never to need to have insulin injections. But it proves the point that endurance exercise such as running is not necessarily something to be avoided by diabetics – it can actually play a big part in helping them to manage and improve their condition.

Running for diabetics

As I mentioned earlier, if you have diabetes, you do need to take extra precautions if you start pushing your body.

One of the first lessons drummed into me was to stretch my legs after I completed my run. I know it's boring, but it will help you avoid injuries and (if you are carrying one) to 'stretch' the scar tissue and speed its recovery. Most people assume that you should do it before you set off – not a good idea unless your legs are already warmed up.

The key muscle groups to concentrate on are your calves, quads (the ones on the front!) and the hamstrings (the ones at the back!).

Stand in a place where you are not going to fall over – put your hand on a fence or wall – and stretch each group on each leg for about 20 seconds, very gradually. Don't 'bounce' your muscles in the stretch as this will be counterproductive.

Check your feet after your run and watch out for blisters and any discomfort. If you do develop any problems, see a state-registered chiropodist. Don't use methyl salicylate or any medication that contains a localised painkiller because this can mask any problems.

Don't forget, if you are on insulin or other medication to take a bum bag, saddle bag or haversack with you containing a blood glucose testing kit, identification, money for emergencies, food, glucose tablets, drinks, etc.

If you are on insulin, as is explained in detail on the Diabetes UK website, "Because insulin is absorbed more rapidly from sites involved in physical activity, before exercising it is best to inject into a site not especially taxed in your activity (the stomach, for example)."

The website goes on to say that it is important to discuss your medication with your diabetes care team, who will advise you on the most appropriate treatment and any changes that need making to your normal regime.

Blood glucose monitoring

If you are someone whose diabetes needs close medical supervision, please read this section carefully. It has been taken directly from the Diabetes UK website. As I have said many times, the exercise regime I adopted has played a big part in getting me where I am today – free of the symptoms. But there are many diabetics out there who have a more serious level of the disease than I did – and if you are going to exercise strenuously, caution has to be the watchword. I'm sure Sir Steve Redgrave must have gone through this or a similar process many times!

- Testing your blood glucose levels before, during and after a training session requires a blood glucose meter that is easy to use while exercising. Keep a record of your readings in a training log, and record details of the distance and time of the session, the food eaten and insulin doses taken so that you can establish a pattern of likely insulin needs and glucose requirements for future sessions. You may also like to discuss these with your diabetes care team.

- Depending on the results of your pre-activity blood glucose test, you may well need to eat some starchy carbohydrate food before you start. If the test shows that your blood glucose level is 13mmol/l or above, you must also test for ketones (test strips are available from your GP). Even if ketones are not present, there may still not be enough insulin for your muscles to be able to mobilise the energy needed to exercise. Your blood glucose level will rise further as a response to the activity and yet, without insulin, still not provide the muscles with energy. Delay the training session until your insulin has taken effect and your blood glucose level has come down.

- If ketones are present, this indicates that fat is being metabolised for energy. If a positive ketone test accompanies a high blood glucose level, this may be a sign of ketoacidosis and you should seek medical help immediately.

- It is important to realise that your body takes up to 36 hours to recover from strenuous activity. The process of muscle refuelling will continue to use up any carbohydrate that is eaten until the muscles are replenished. Be aware of the risk of hypos – not only overnight but also the following day. Have a bedtime snack and monitor your blood glucose level when you wake.

- If you are going to start upping your mileage, you will

probably find that you need to increase your portions of starchy carbohydrate foods at all meals and snacks during the training period, as well as reducing your insulin dose. (As I said, exercise allows you to take a few more liberties with your diet). Eating plenty of starchy carbohydrate foods not only helps prevent hypos, it also helps replenish stores of energy in the muscles after each training session.

- Research suggests that eating a combination of protein and carbohydrate increases the uptake of muscle glycogen, while food eaten within two hours of activity promotes maximum intake into the muscles and liver. Muscles that are well nourished are less prone to injury and more responsive to training, so it is worth adjusting your eating times to fit in with your next training session.

- During any training session lasting more than one hour it is important to take more carbohydrate and fluids. Fluids which also contain carbohydrate are useful, eg fruit juice and squash, or isotonic sports drinks. During a long or strenuous ride or run, eat more carbohydrate snacks, such as sports bars, cereal bars, chocolate or bananas.

- If you have been swimming... you may feel hungrier afterwards than you would do had you done some other kind of sport. This is because of the extra calorific effort involved in maintaining body temperature, whilst also using calories to produce energy. Having a carbohydrate snack straight after swimming can begin the resynthesis of muscle glycogen that is necessary to keep you in good condition.

- Drink plenty of water during and after the training session. Thirst is a sign of dehydration. Drink small amounts frequently, even if you are not thirsty – approximately 150ml of fluid every 15 minutes - because dehydration dramatically affects performance.

- Isotonic sports drinks, typically, contain 5-8 g per 100 ml. of quickly absorbed carbohydrates which can help to give the blood glucose level a boost during strenuous exercise. Sports drinks do not cause delayed stomach emptying or stomach cramps and can be used before and during a race. This is in contrast to drinks with more than 8g of, carbohydrate per 100 mls, which can cause stomach cramps and slow down fluid absorption due to their effects of delaying stomach emptying. These drinks, eg Red Bull, Purdeys, Lipovitan, B3 and Power House, are not recommended.

Chapter 7
The next steps

"I have put my diabetes behind me. I'm on no medication whatsoever – including the blood pressure tablets that pre-dated my diabetes. I'm not going to risk either condition returning by being silly about my diet again. And, to be honest, there's no need to."

Well as I've mentioned, I started off at around 15 stone (210 pounds), at the beginning of 2009. I'm now 11 stone, I have been for many months, and fully intending to stay around that weight. It may not be the right weight for everyone: I've always been wiry rather than muscular – the extra four stone was just masking that!

I am quite happy to allow that to creep up by a few pounds from time to time, but I will never let myself get back into the position, or the physical state, that I was in. I really enjoy being this weight – I bounce up stairs rather than feeling that I've got a sack of potatoes weighing me down. And that's what four stone or 56 pounds is: a bag of spuds!

And talking of spuds, I can tuck into my biggest single treat of the week - a big plate of cod and chips (with mushy peas) every Saturday lunchtime – with a completely clear conscience. If a few ounces do go on, they will soon come off again.

Critically, I have put my diabetes behind me. I'm on no mediation whatsoever – including the blood pressure tablets that pre-dated my diabetes. I'm not going to risk either condition returning by being silly about my diet again. And, to be honest, there's no need to. I have got into a routine of eating delicious food which also happens to be healthy. I have increased my food intake to allow for the exercise I am taking, and have yet to suffer any symptoms associated with running out of energy. I can get away with an odd treat with no ill effects at all.

It's plain that my body is working effectively again. I also weigh myself using an accurate pair of scales every morning, so I have a complete handle on what my body is doing – and that is important.

From here, I plan to keep up a sensible regime of eating and exercise that will keep me healthy – and you can too. I certainly intend to carry on running, and have set my sights on a sub 1.50 time in the next Cardiff half marathon, and a sub 55 in the next 10k race.

I don't think that what I've achieved defies medical science. It simply proves that, if you give it some help, the body does have the ability to mend itself. I would never claim that this diet and exercise regime will have such a dramatic effect with people on insulin injections, or whose organs have been permanently damaged. But everything I have read persuades me that it can make a difference, perhaps an important difference, to a lot of people.

I am also convinced that echoing what I did could have a massively beneficial effect on those half a million people currently walking around with early stages of diabetes, and which has not yet been diagnosed. And to the millions whose blood sugar is too high and who are putting their long term health at risk. It may even help them avoid succumbing to the full blown version of the disease by getting their food intake back down to a point where it matches its 'output'.

And I am even more confident that anyone out there who is carrying more weight than they want or need to have will find this diet as effective and enjoyable as any currently being promoted.

As I have made plain, it will require some willpower – but not as much as the diets that leave you hungry, or gnawing on food that you find boring and tasteless. The results are quick and, I at least never hit a wall, after which the pounds stubbornly refused to budge. Moreover, it is based on sound science.

So why not give it a go?

Over the following pages my wife Bev and I have set out some of the recipes that have made this year one of the best I have ever had for eating. Do I miss those late night curries? Of course I do. But as the suggestions on eating out make plain, you still can enjoy great foreign cuisine – by selecting the right items off the menu.

So enjoy – and I hope to see you at the line up of a race in the not too distant future. I'll be the one proudly wearing a Diabetes UK Cymru top!

The recipes & diet plan

"Missing breakfast is common, but not smart. Many people believe that they will lose weight if they skip meals, but this is not true. To reverse my diabetes and lose weight, while still doing a hard day's work, my body needed to be refuelled five times each day - starting with a good healthy, filling breakfast."

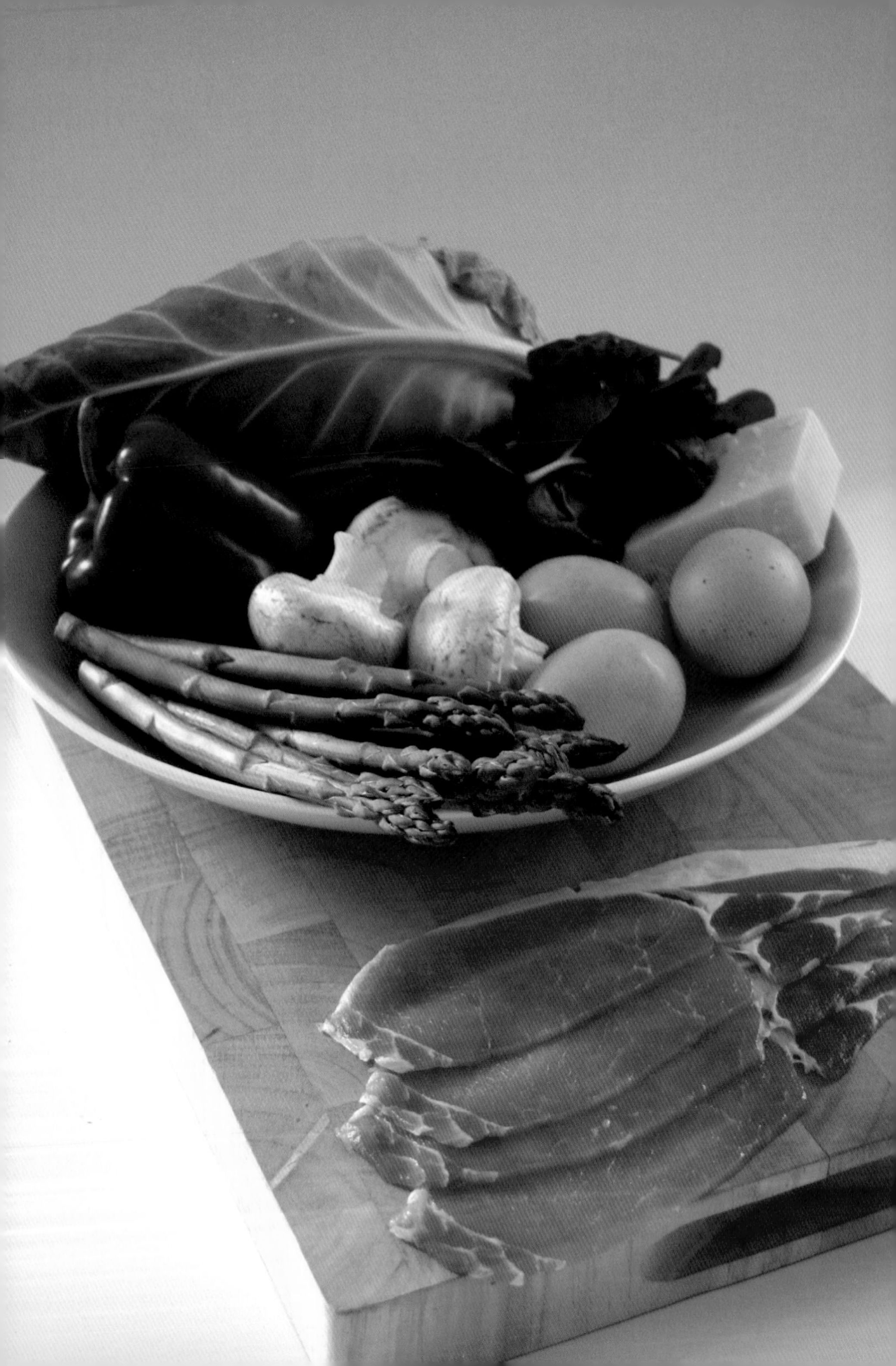

Breakfast

Choice of ingredients

Eggs
Bacon
Cheese (low fat)
Green peppers
Asparagus
Spinach
Mushrooms
Sweetheart cabbage
Onion
Extra virgin olive oil

Equipment

Egg poacher
Small frying pan
12 cup deep muffin tin
Paper baking cups

Missing breakfast is common, but not smart. Many people believe that they will lose weight if they skip meals, but this is not true. To reverse my diabetes and lose weight, while still doing a hard day's work, my body needed to be refuelled five times each day - starting with a good healthy, filling breakfast.

Breakfast recipes

Asparagus, mushroom & spinach omelette

2 medium eggs; 3 asparagus spears; 1 medium sized mushroom – sliced
1 tablespoon olive oil; 200g/8oz fresh spinach
Cut asparagus into pieces. Heat olive oil in pan, add asparagus and sauté until tender. Add spinach, sauté for a couple more minutes. Pour in egg mixture and sliced mushroom. Cook omelette for 1 minute. When the top starts to firm up, using a turner, flip the omelette over. Cook for a further 20-30 seconds or so until each side is a very light golden brown.

Poached egg & bacon

1 fresh egg & 2 slices lean bacon
Fill the pan with 1 inch of water. Bring to a boil. Lightly coat one poacher egg cup with olive oil, crack egg into cup. Cover and all to cook for 3-4 minutes. Grill/fry bacon.

Poached egg with sautéed cabbage & spinach

Poach egg as above.
2 tablespoons extra virgin olive oil ; 200g/8oz fresh Spinach; 200g/8oz sweetheart cabbage
Shred cabbage. Heat the oil, add cabbage, sauté until tender and turning golden brown. Add the spinach and sauté for a couple more minutes.

Quiche bites

300g/10 oz frozen spinach, 1 bunch spring onions finely chopped
4 eggs, beaten; 450g/16 oz low fat cottage cheese; 225g/8 oz grated low fat cheese
Preheat oven to 160°c/Gas mark 3. Set up baking tray with pre-oiled round paper baking cups. Place spinach in a small saucepan. Cook over medium heat, stirring occasionally until soft. Drain off any remaining liquid. Stir in spring onions, eggs, cottage cheese and cheddar cheese. Pour mixture into as many baking cups as quantity will allow. Bake uncovered in preheated oven for 45-60 minutes, until eggs are set. Freeze remainder for future use.

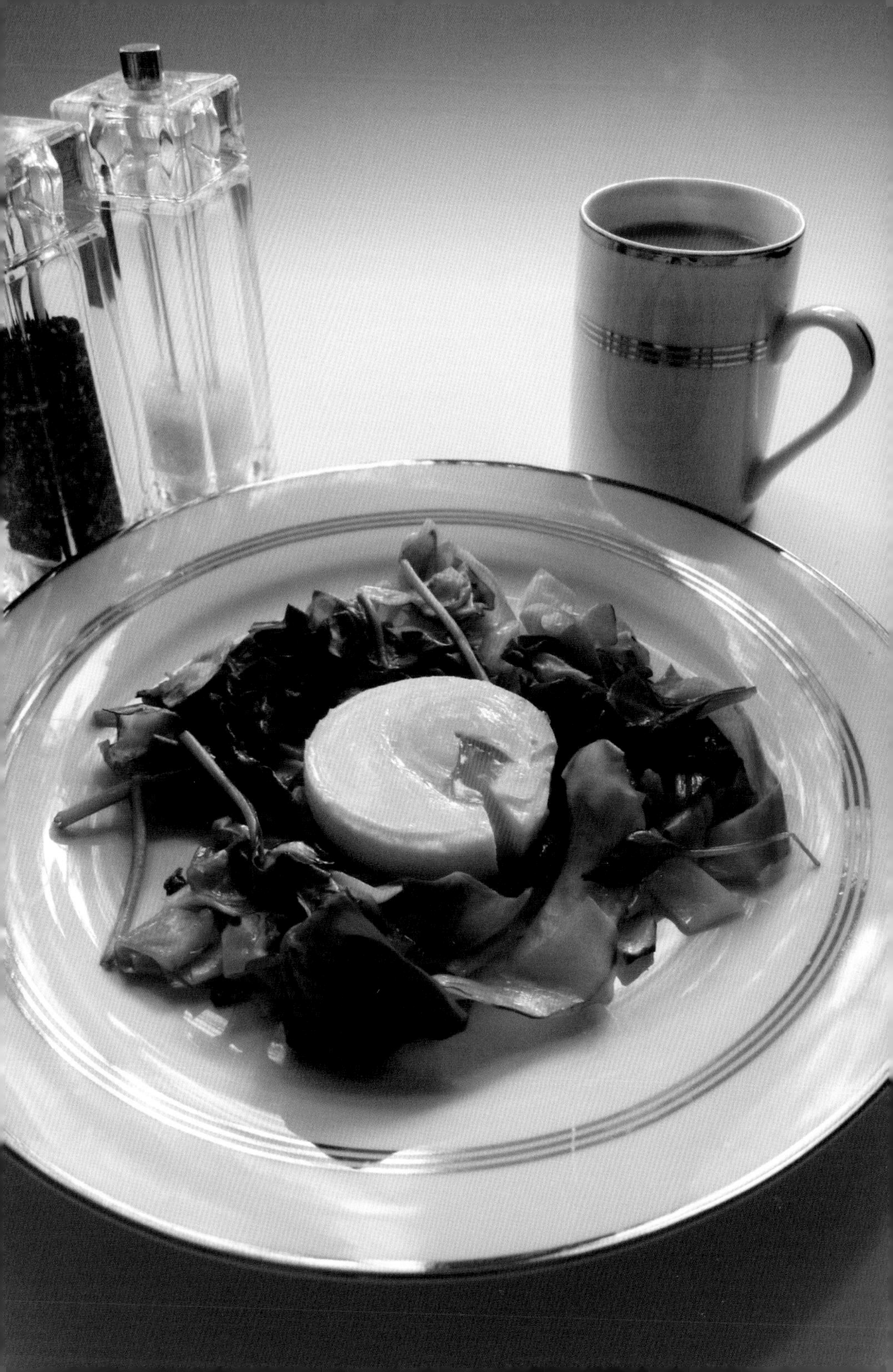

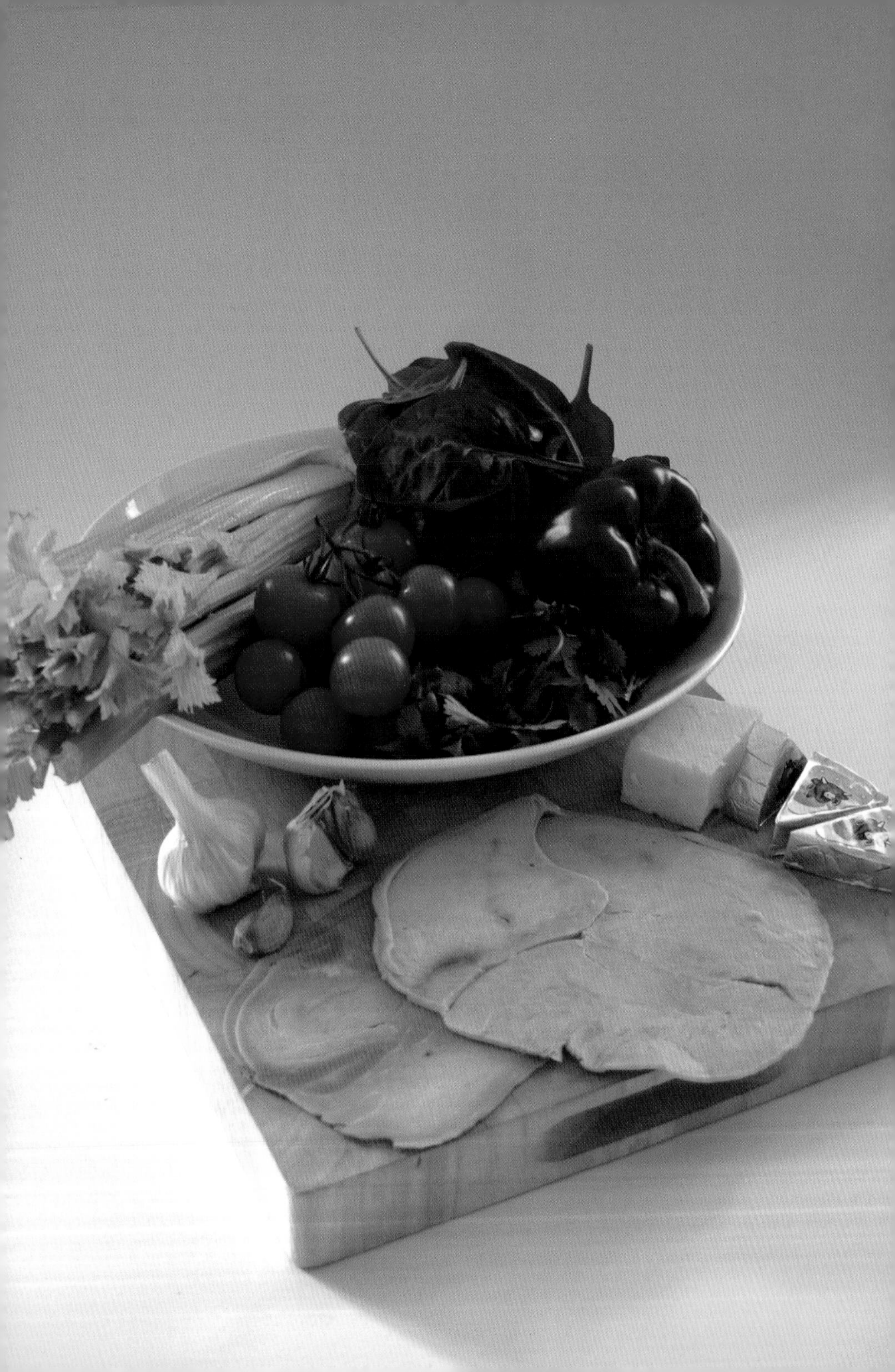

Mid morning/afternoon snacks

Choice of ingredients

Sliced cooked chicken
Sliced cooked turkey
Sliced cooked ham
Celery
Cherry/Plum tomatoes
Spinach
Green peppers
Low fat cheese spread
Lettuce
Cheese (low fat)

Herbs:
Basil
Coriander
Dill
Garlic
Rosemary

Mid morning/afternoon snacks - a must in a daily diet. Only 2 to 3 hours after breakfast and lunch and you eat again- this is essential for you to keep away the hunger pangs and, at the same time, take on board some key ingredients to break down those sugars in your system. Take these with you wrapped in cling film to eat on the fly!

Mid morning/afternoon snack recipes

Wraps

Ham
Spread low fat mayo on a slice of cooked ham; layer with spinach leaves, sprinkle with coriander leaves; roll and hold secure with cocktail stick.

Chicken
As above – substitute slice of cooked chicken breast for ham

Turkey
As above – substitute slice of cooked turkey breast for chicken

Cheese chunk & tomatoes

A 3oz chunk of low fat Cheddar cheese with 6 small plum tomatoes

Celery with cheese spread & olives

Fill the celery stalk with low fat soft cheese spread and eat with six green or black olives

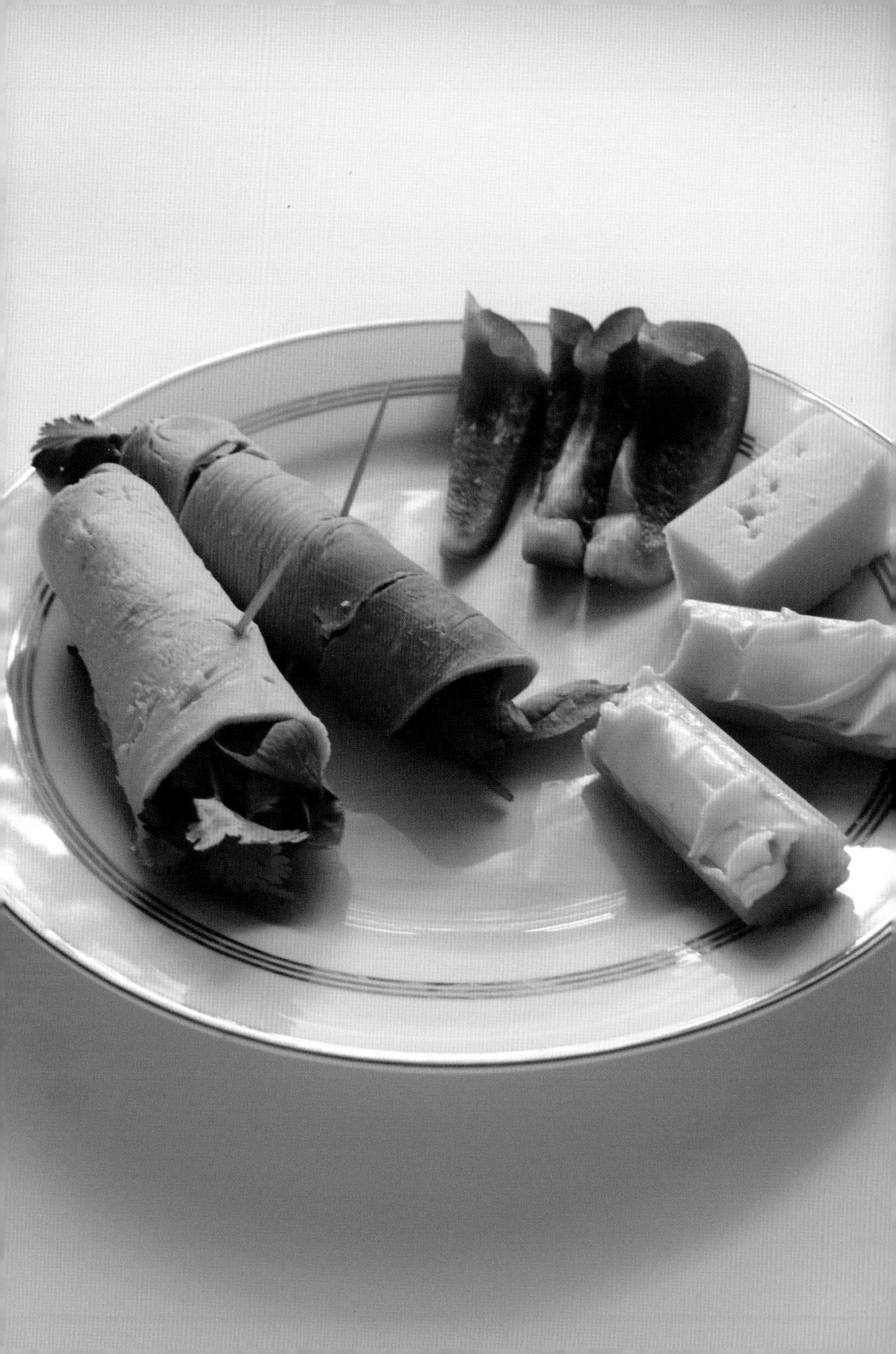

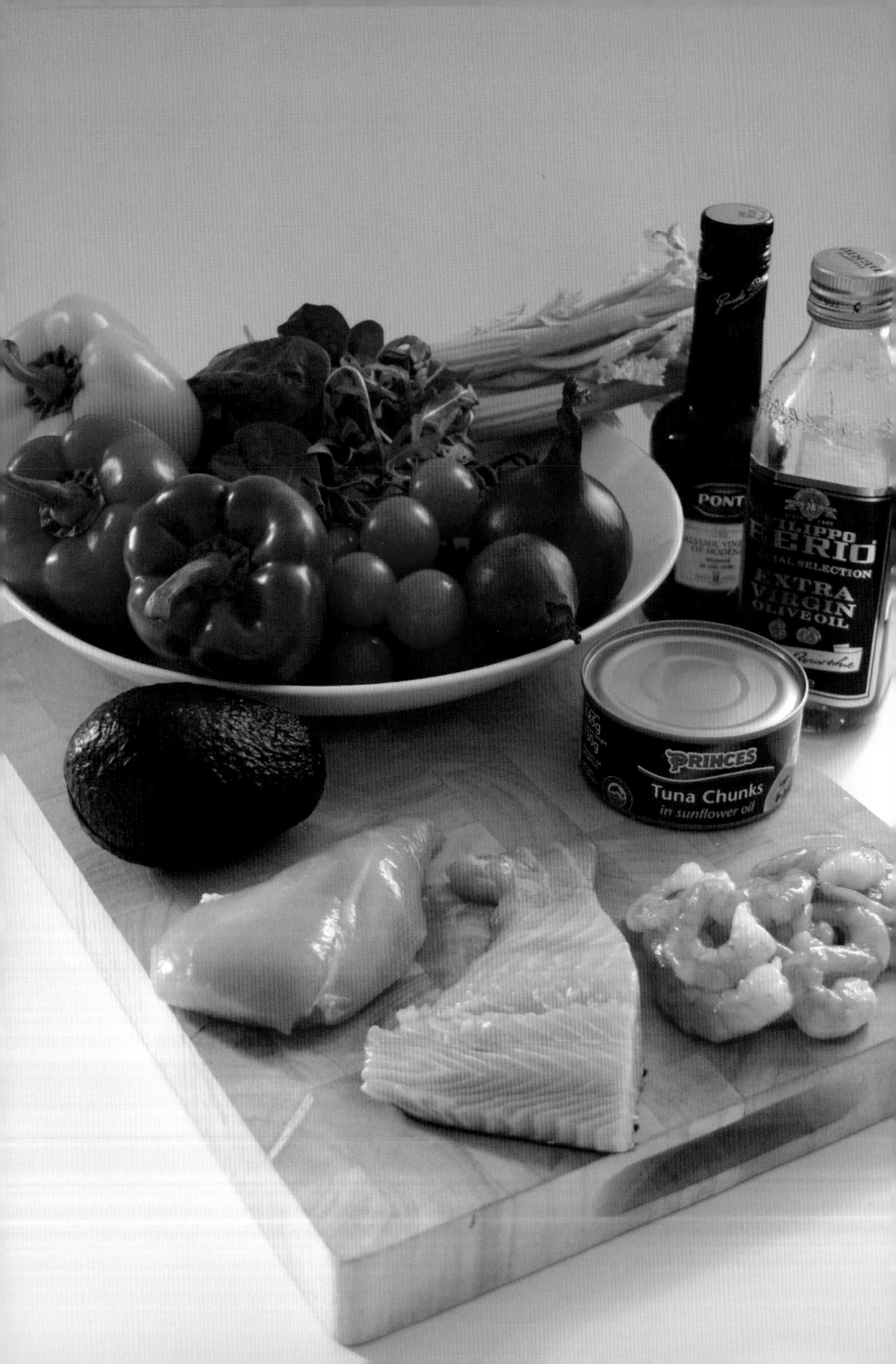
EXTRA
VIRGIN
OLIVE OIL
PRINCES
Tuna Chunks
in sunflower oil

Lunch

Choice of ingredients

Chicken breast
Tuna (tinned or fresh)
Salmon (tinned or fresh)
Cooked prawns
Sliced beef

Salad:
Celery
Lettuce
Spinach
Tomatoes
Peppers red, green, yellow
Avocado
Spring onions
Red onions
Dressing

Equipment

George Foreman grill

Lunch - for me an air-tight plastic container full! Try and have this just after midday if you can (unless you are on shifts) as leaving it late will create a 'domino' effect on your dinner - and you shouldn't eat that too late!

Lunch recipes

Chicken breast/beef burger with mixed salad

1 skinless, boneless chicken breast/beef burger

Grill chicken breast/beef burger for 7 minutes until completely done after seasoning with salt, pepper and a spray of extra virgin olive oil.

Salmon fillet with mixed salad

1 salmon fillet

Coat grill with spray of extra virgin olive oil. Place salmon fillet skin side down on grill. Grill, covered, over medium-hot heat for 12-15 minutes or until fish flakes easily with a fork. Cover and eat cold.

Tinned salmon with mixed salad

Mash a tin of Princes/ John West Salmon together with Hellmans Light mayo. Add 1 chopped celery stalk and half a red onion (optional).

Tuna steak with mixed salad

1 tuna steak

Grill tuna on the grill for just 2-3 minutes. The tuna should be quite pink in the middle.

Tinned tuna with mixed salad

Mash a tin of Princes/ John West Tuna in spring water together with Hellmans Light mayo. Add 1 chopped celery stalk and half a red onion (optional).

King prawn with mixed salad

Half of a 225g pack of Tesco cooked, peeled king prawns

Large mixed salad bowl

Rub cold salad bowl with cut garlic. Break a crisp, dry lettuce and a packet of spinach leaves into bowl. Add 15 cherry tomatoes on top, then add red onions, sliced thin. Chop up and add a green, red & yellow pepper. Sprinkle with parsley and chill at least a half hour before serving. Add any low fat dressing of your choice.

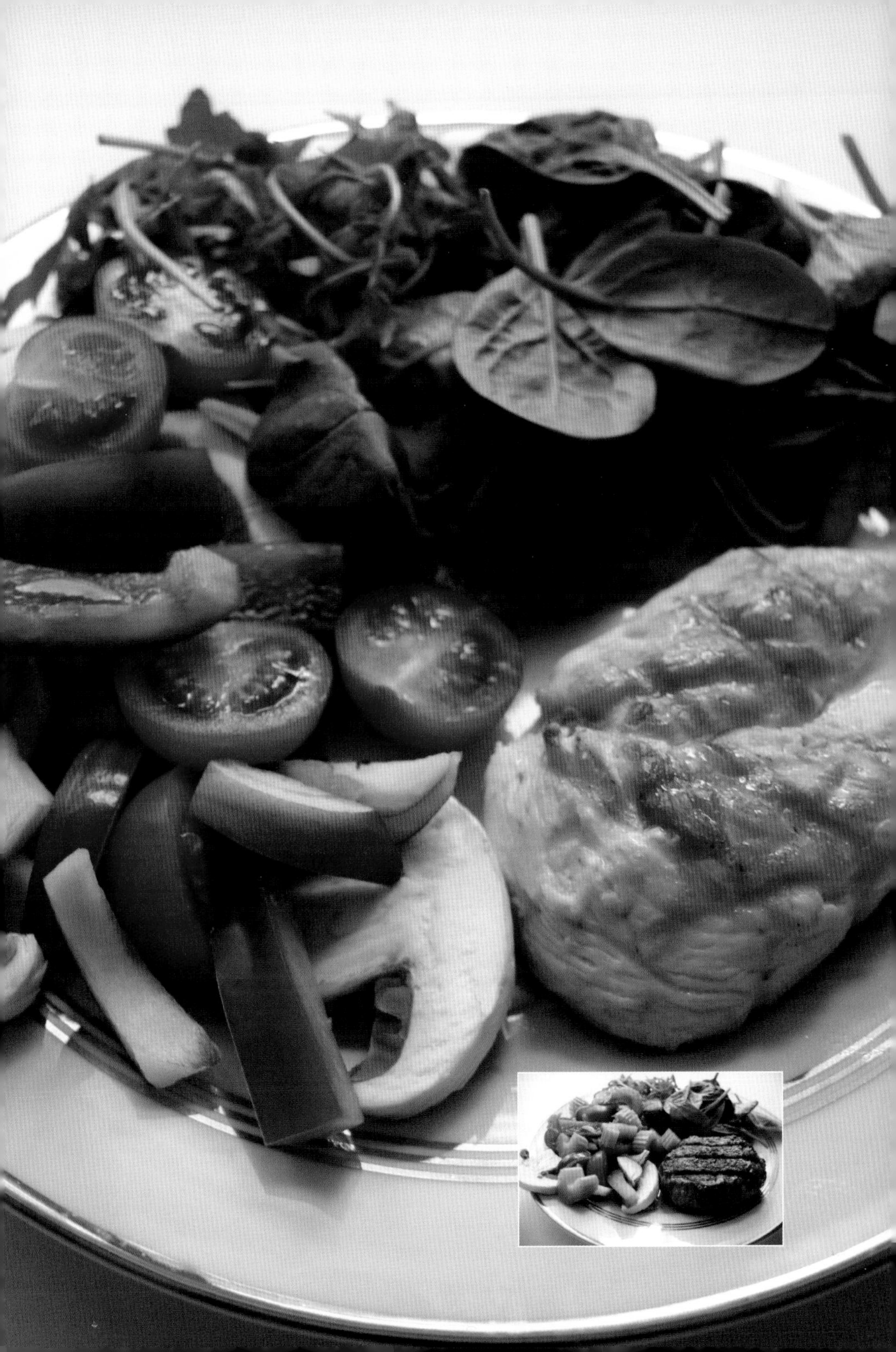

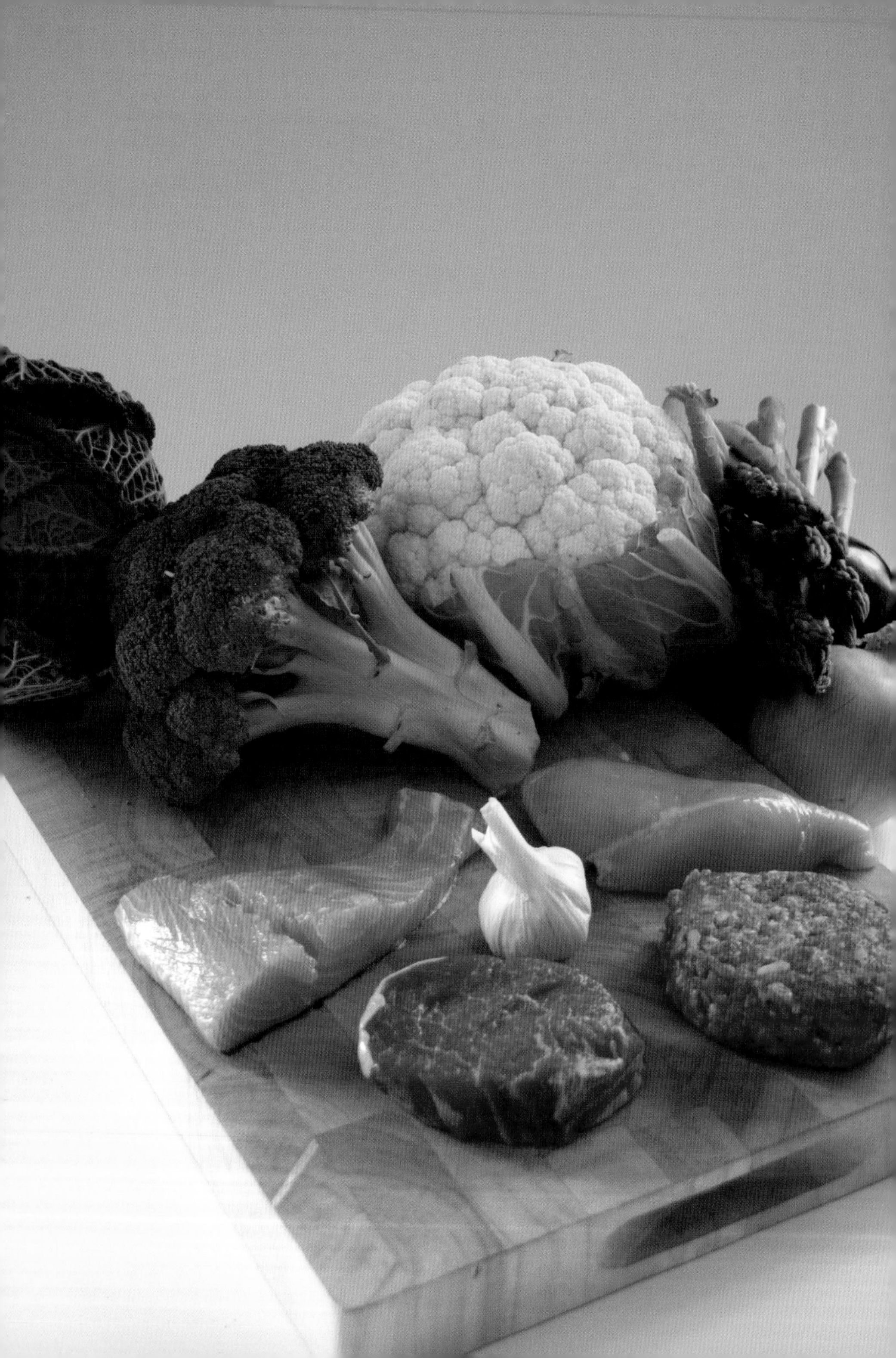

Dinner

Choice of ingredients

Meat:
Chicken breast
Beef burgers
Steak

Fish:
Tuna steak
Salmon fillet
Bream
Cod fillet
Coley
Hake
Red snapper
Smoked haddock
Swordfish
Trout
King prawns
Lobster

Vegetables:
Asparagus
Broccoli
Cabbage
Cauliflower
Leeks
Broad beans

Salad:
Celery
Spinach
Lettuce
Peppers red, green, yellow
Red onions
Spinach
Spring onions
Tomatoes
Dressing

Equipment
George Foreman grill
Conventional oven
Stainless steel 3-piece steamer

To think, it was only three hours before that you have a mid afternoon snack and now you're going to have a big meal! Mashed cauliflower and plenty of vegetables with your meat or fish is a good way to fill yourself up here: eat as much as you like of these, but remember to eat at least a few hours before you go to bed.

Dinner recipes

Baked salmon with prawns, leek & asparagus

1 salmon fillet; 225 frozen uncooked peeled prawns; 5/6 asparagus spears; 1 leek

Peel onion, cut in half, slice thickly. Arrange the onion slices on a piece of kitchen foil. Spray with olive oil. Place salmon fillet on top. Sprinkle fresh dill, season and close foil packet. Place on oven tray and bake until cooked through, about 25-30 minutes on 190°c/gas mark 5. Wash and trim 5/6 asparagus spears, steam for 6-8 minutes until tender. Peel and cut the leek into rings and steam for 5-7 minutes. Season and add squeeze of fresh lemon juice. Five minutes before the asparagus is ready, add half of a 225g packet of uncooked, peeled, frozen prawns to the water in the base of steamer and cook until they turn pink. Place the prawns on top of salmon, arrange the asparagus and leeks.

Baked chicken & roasted vegetables

Skinless, boneless chicken breast; 6 small white onions; quarter cup of dry white wine; 1 chicken stock cube; 2 garlic cloves, minced; Juice of half of a fresh lemon; 1 teaspoon tarragon

Spray a baking dish with olive oil spray. Heat oven to 190°c/gas mark 5. Arrange chicken in baking dish with peeled onions. Combine wine, stock cube, garlic, lemon juice, and tarragon; pour over chicken. Season with salt, pepper. Bake for 20 minutes. Baste and bake for 15 minutes longer, or until chicken is cooked through and browned. In a large bowl combine diced green, red & yellow pepper, red onion quartered and diced celery with 4 tablespoons of olive oil, two tablespoons of balsamic vinegar, two tablespoons of chopped fresh rosemary and one crushed garlic clove. Stir well to make sure all vegetables are coated and spread evenly onto an oven tray. roast for 25-30 minutes at 190°c/gas mark 5.

Grilled fillet steak with cauli mash & tomatoes

Large fillet steak, small cauliflower & 4 tomatoes

Coat grill rack with spray of extra virgin olive oil. Place fillet steak on grill. Grill, covered, over medium-hot heat for 8-10 minutes turning once. Steam a small cauli until really tender. Add to blender with a large spoonful of Benecol/Flora light. Blend until consistency resembles mashed potatoes. Serve cauli mash with grilled tomatoes.

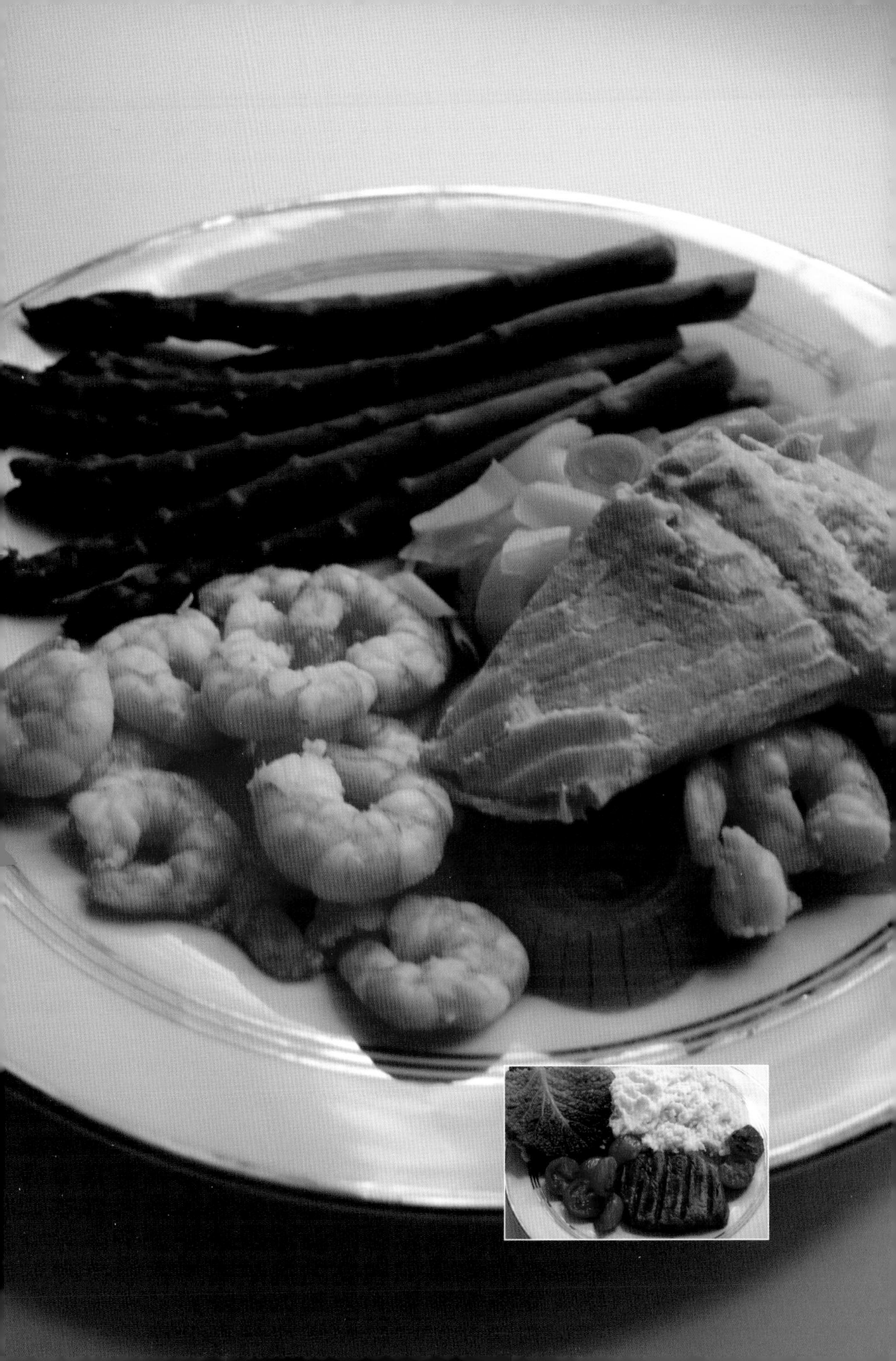

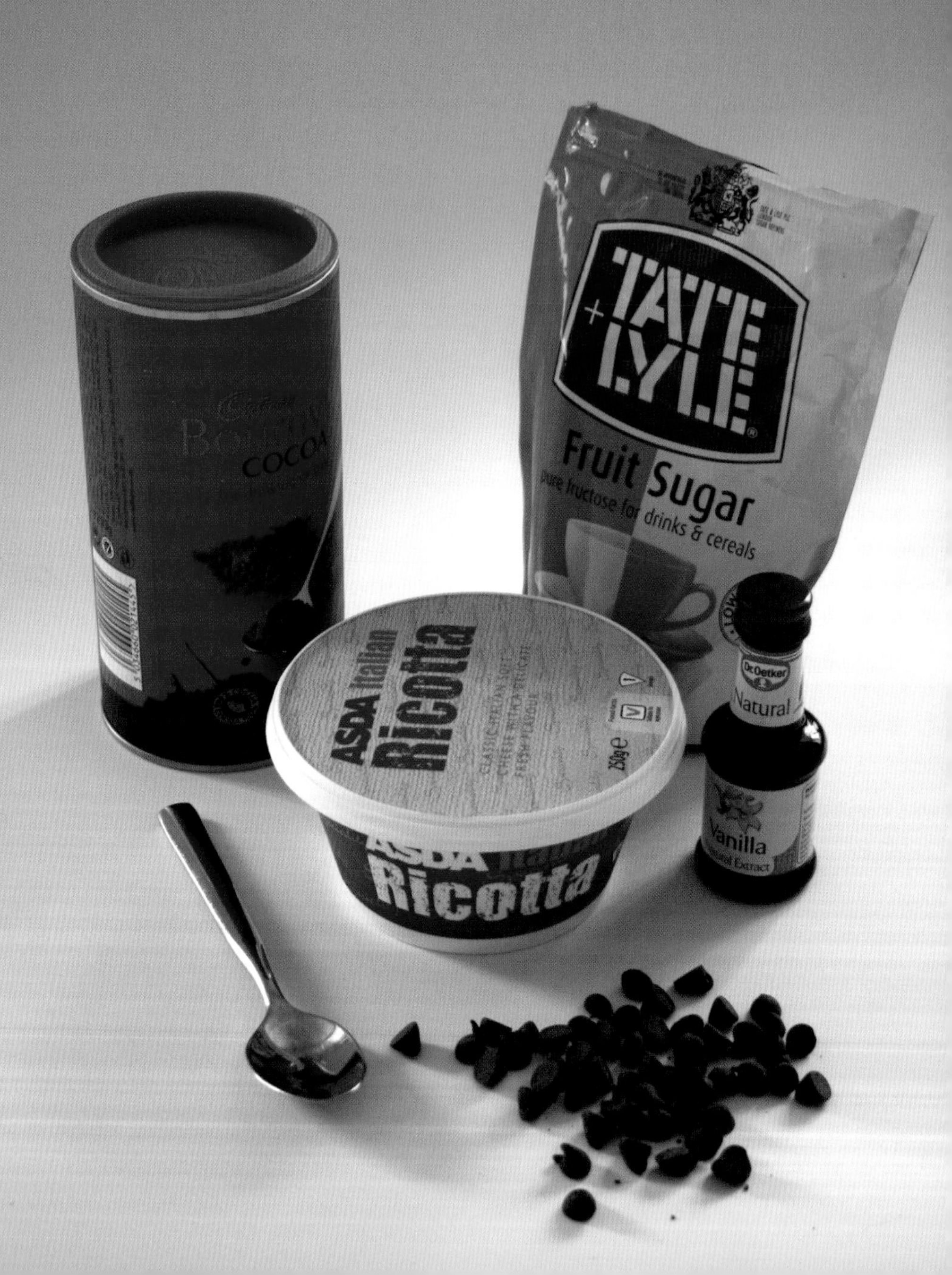
COCOA
TATE + LYLE
Fruit Sugar
pure fructose for drinks & cereals
ASDA Italian
Ricotta
CLASSIC ITALIAN SOFT CHEESE WITH A DELICATE FRESH FLAVOUR
250g
Dr.Oetker
Natural
Vanilla
Natural Extract

Desserts

Ingredients

Ricotta cheese
Fruit sugar
Vanilla essence
Chocolate chip chunks
Low calorie jelly
Low fat custard
Rhubarb
Prunes

Equipment

Heavy based saucepan

Chocolate? On a diet? How does that work? Well it did with me. I had ricotta with (a modest amount of) cocoa and chocolate chips after the main meal just about every night - and I still managed to lose weight, lower my blood pressure and reverse my diabetes. Bliss!

Dessert recipes

Lemon ricotta
Half a 250g tub Asda/Walmart ricotta cheese
1 tablespoon of freshly squeezed lemon juice
Lemon zest
1 teaspoon vanilla essence
2 teaspoon Tate & Lyle fruit sugar [to taste]

Place essence, sugar and lemon juice into chilled serving dish. Add ricotta cheese and mix vigorously for 10-15 seconds. Sprinkle in a teaspoon of lemon zest.

Chocolate ricotta
Half a 250g tub Asda/Walmart ricotta cheese
1 tablespoon of 1-2 teaspoons Cadburys cocoa powder
1 teaspoon vanilla essence
1 teaspoon Tate & Lyle fruit sugar [to taste]
Plain chocolate chips

Place essence, sugar, cocoa into chilled serving dish. Add ricotta cheese and mix vigorously for 10-15 seconds. Sprinkle in a handful of dark [or milk] chocolate chips and add several to top as decoration.

Rhubarb & custard
Fresh rhubarb
150g pot of Ambrosia low fat Devon custard
2 teaspoon Tate & Lyle fruit sugar

Wash and cut the rhubarb into bite size pieces, place into a heavy-based saucepan, pour in enough water to cover the rhubarb, then cook over a low heat for 10 minutes - stirring occasionally. Remove from heat and allow to cool and serve with custard.

Prunes & custard
Tinned prunes in prune juice (not in syrup)
150g pot of Ambrosia low fat Devon custard

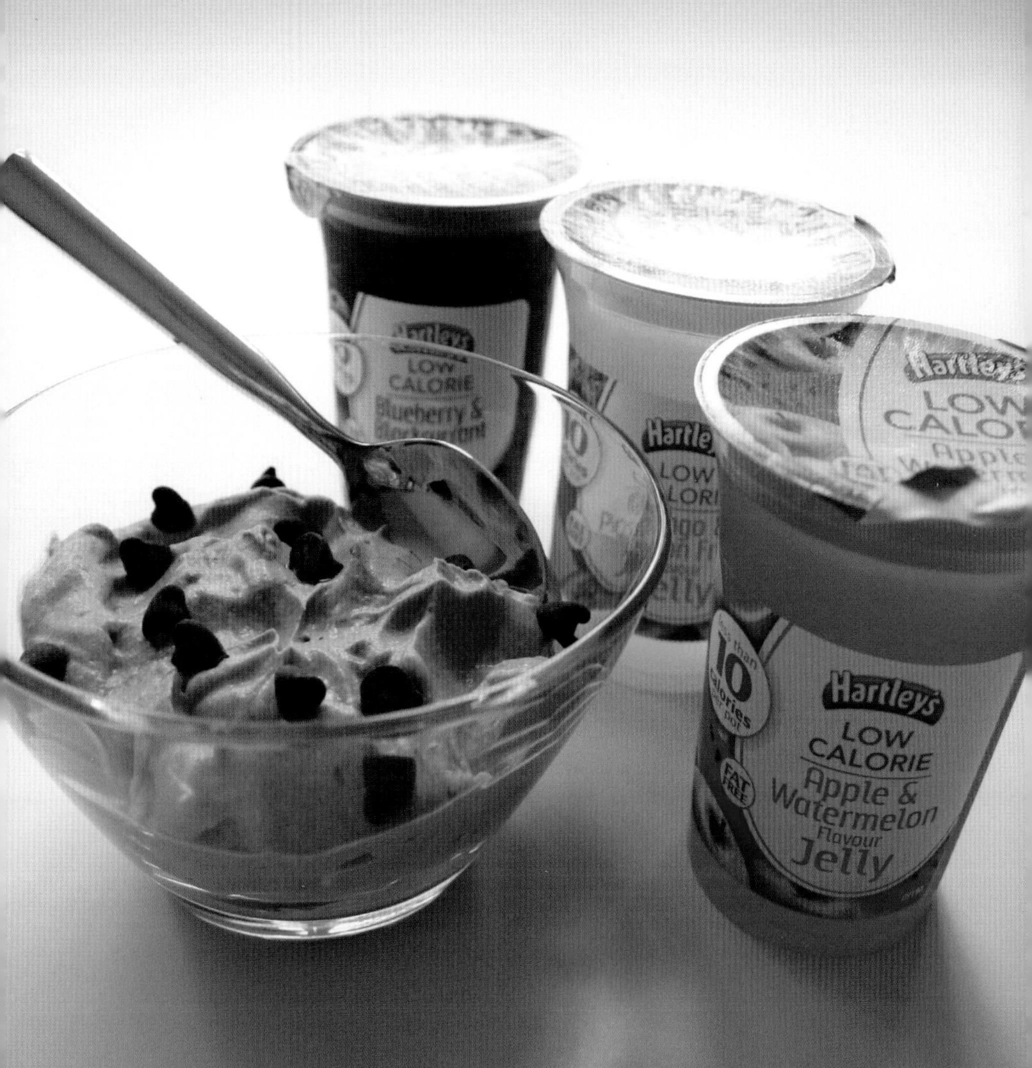
Hartley's
LOW
CALORIE
Blueberry &
Hartley's
LOW
10
calories
Hartley's
LOW
CALORIE
Apple &
Watermelon
Flavour
Jelly
FAT
FREE

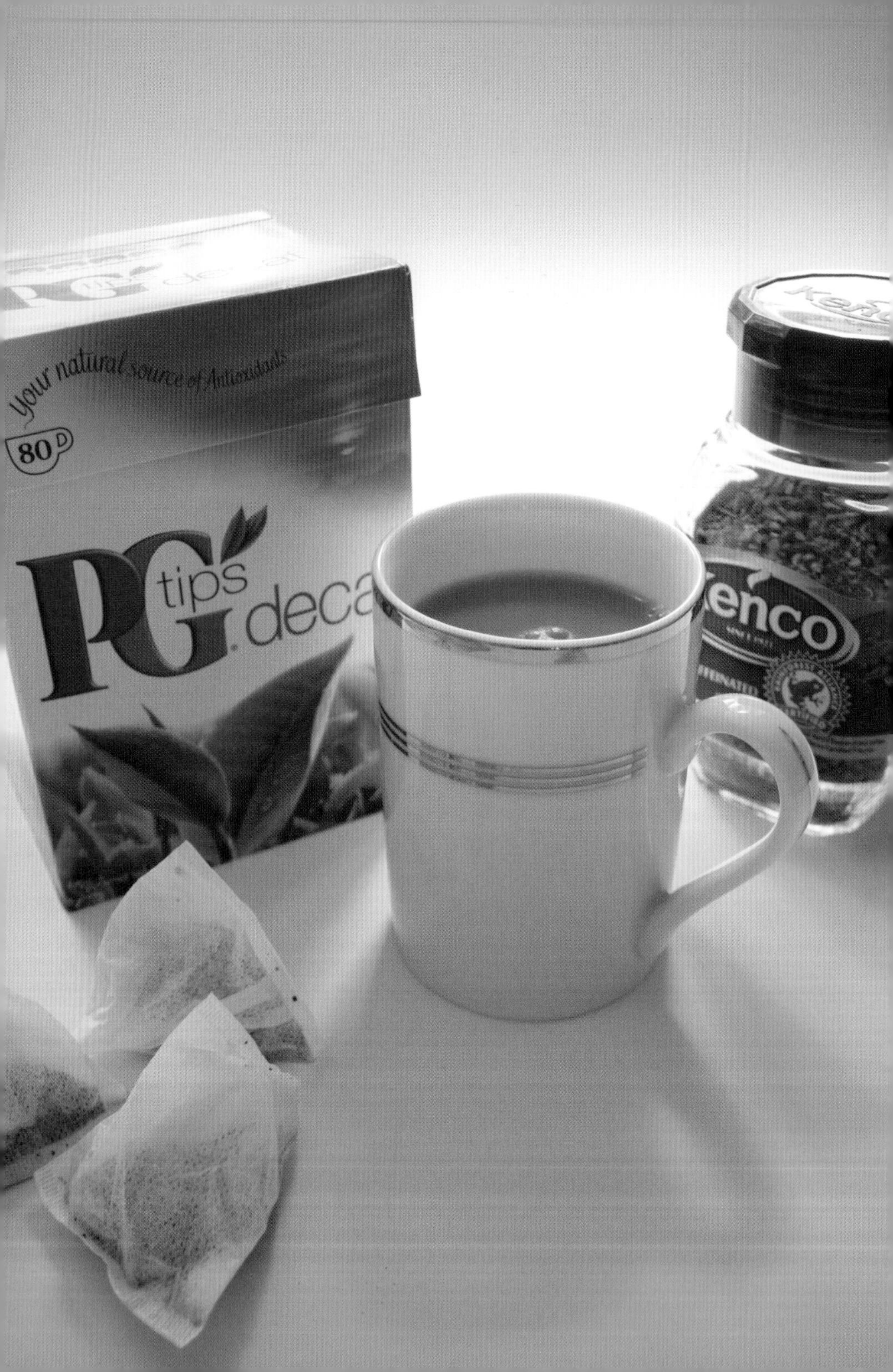
your natural source of Antioxidants
80
PG tips
Kenco

Drinks

Tea - decaf
Coffee - decaf
Water - tap or bottled
Milk - skimmed
Spring water & blackcurrant juice
Water

Vodka & cranberry juice, ice with a slice of lime
(No alcohol in the first month)

Have a cup of tea or coffee (ideally decaf) every morning to wash down the breakfast and set you up for the day, then stick to water.

If you're like me and not keen on just water, get sparkling water and add some low sugar blackcurrant squash such as Ribena. Try to use skimmed milk in your tea and coffee.

Try to steer clear of alcohol to start, but after a month, try a tipple of vodka diet cranberry: an acquired taste but, after a while, you will enjoy it - and the vodka contains no sugar while cranberries have moderate levels of vitamin C, dietary fibre and the essential mineral, manganese.

Restricting alcohol to Friday and Saturday only is a good thing - a discipline I am sticking to even today!

Meal plan day 1

Breakfast

Poached egg with sautéed cabbage & spinach

Mid Morning Snack

Turkey wrap

Lunch

Tuna steak with mixed salad

Mid Afternoon Snack

Ham wrap

Evening Meal

Grilled fillet steak with cauli mash & tomatoes
Ricotta cheese with chocolate

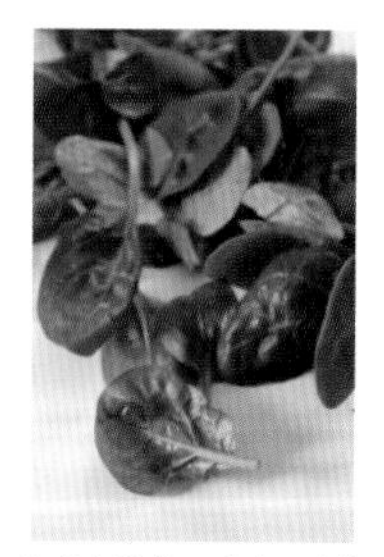

Spinach is rich in vitamins A, C, E & K and should be a key part of a daily diet

Meal plan day 2

Breakfast

Asparagus, mushroom & spinach omelette

Mid Morning Snack

Cheese chunk & tomatoes

Lunch

Chicken breast with mixed salad

Mid Afternoon Snack

Ham wrap

Evening Meal

Baked salmon with prawns, leek & asparagus
Lemon ricotta

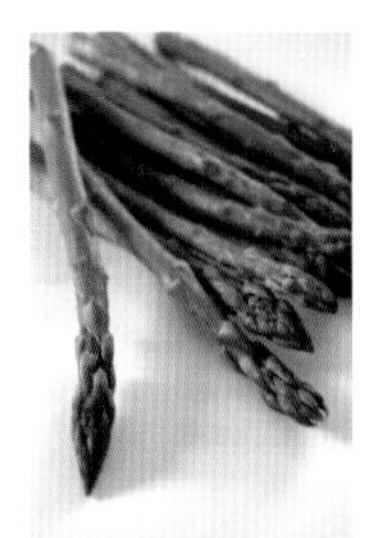

Asparagus is a low-calorie source of folate and potassium

Meal plan day 3

Breakfast

Poached egg & bacon

Mid Morning Snack

Celery with cheese spread & olives

Lunch

Salmon fillet with mixed salad

Mid Afternoon Snack

Ham wrap

Evening Meal

Baked chicken & roasted vegetables
Low calorie jelly

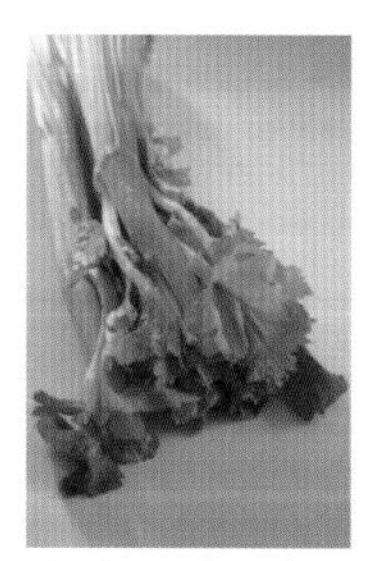

Celery provides low-calorie dietary fibre bulk

Meal plan day 4

Breakfast

Quiche bites

Mid Morning Snack

Chicken wrap

Lunch

King prawn with mixed salad

Mid Afternoon Snack

Cheese chunk & tomatoes

Evening Meal

Grilled fillet steak with cauli mash & tomatoes
Chocolate ricotta

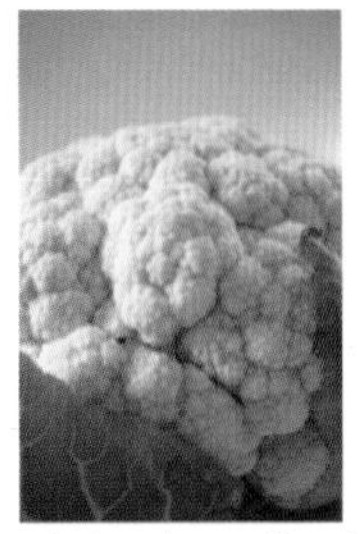

Cauliflower is low in fat, but high in dietary fibre, folate, water and vitamin C

Meal plan day 5

Breakfast

Asparagus, cheese & spinach omelette

Mid Morning Snack

Ham wrap

Lunch

Sliced beef with mixed salad

Mid Afternoon Snack

Turkey wrap

Evening Meal

Baked chicken & roasted vegetables
Low calorie jelly

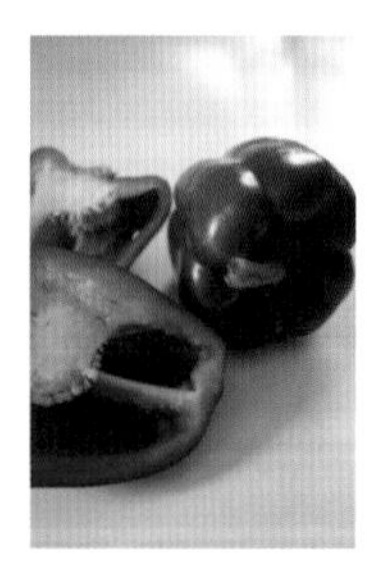

Green peppers are a very good source of fibre, folate, and vitamin K

Meal plan day 6

Breakfast

Boiled eggs

Mid Morning Snack

Cheese chunk & tomatoes

Lunch

Beef burger with mixed salad

Mid Afternoon Snack

Chicken wrap

Evening Meal

Baked salmon with prawns, leek & asparagus
Rhubarb & custard

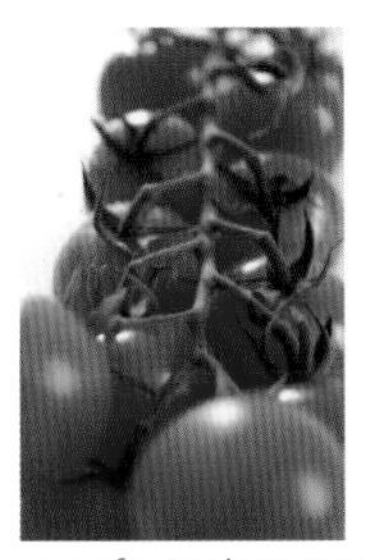

Tomatoes contain lycopene, one of nature's most powerful natural antioxidants

Meal plan day 7

Breakfast

Poached egg & bacon with fried tomatoes

Mid Morning Snack

Turkey wrap

Lunch

Salmon fillet with mixed salad

Mid Afternoon Snack

Celery with cheese spread & olives

Evening Meal

Grilled fillet steak with cauli mash & broccoli
Low calorie jelly

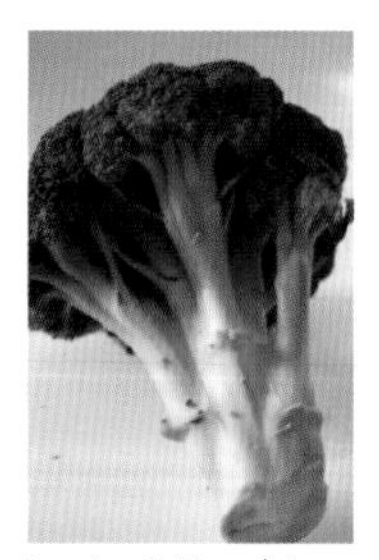

Broccoli is high in vitamins C, K, and A, as well as dietary fibre

Eating Out

If you are anything like me, you'll enjoy going out for a meal after a hard day's work or to celebrate a special occasion – or just it being the weekend. You may think that restaurants don't do diet food - unless it's a salad! Not true. If you go out with family or friends, you really don't have to be the 'odd one out'. Just be selective. And here are a few ideas.

Indian meals can have huge calorie counts. But a lot of the problem is the sauces. Always go for something without a sauce (for instance, the Tandoori items) and stay away from the pappadoms and naan breads! My personal favorite is Lamb or King Prawn Tikka, and this normally comes with a side salad, but I always complement the meal with a Saag Bhaji: spinach stir fried with onions and herbs - delicious!

Chinese meals also need caution because, once again, the sauces are rich in unwanted carbs. But there are some great foods you can have with a clear conscience. My favourite is Fu Yung - a type of a thick omelette with beansprouts and either prawns or chicken.

Steak houses - You can really go for it here with a nice lean, grilled steak or, better still, the grilled fish that many steak houses offer. Just watch out for the fries or jacket potatoes that usually go with them – load up on salad instead, dressed with olive oil and balsamic vinegar. If someone else complains about you not eating chips – let them have yours!

Remember - carbs are only 'on your side' if you are the ideal weight and doing exercise.

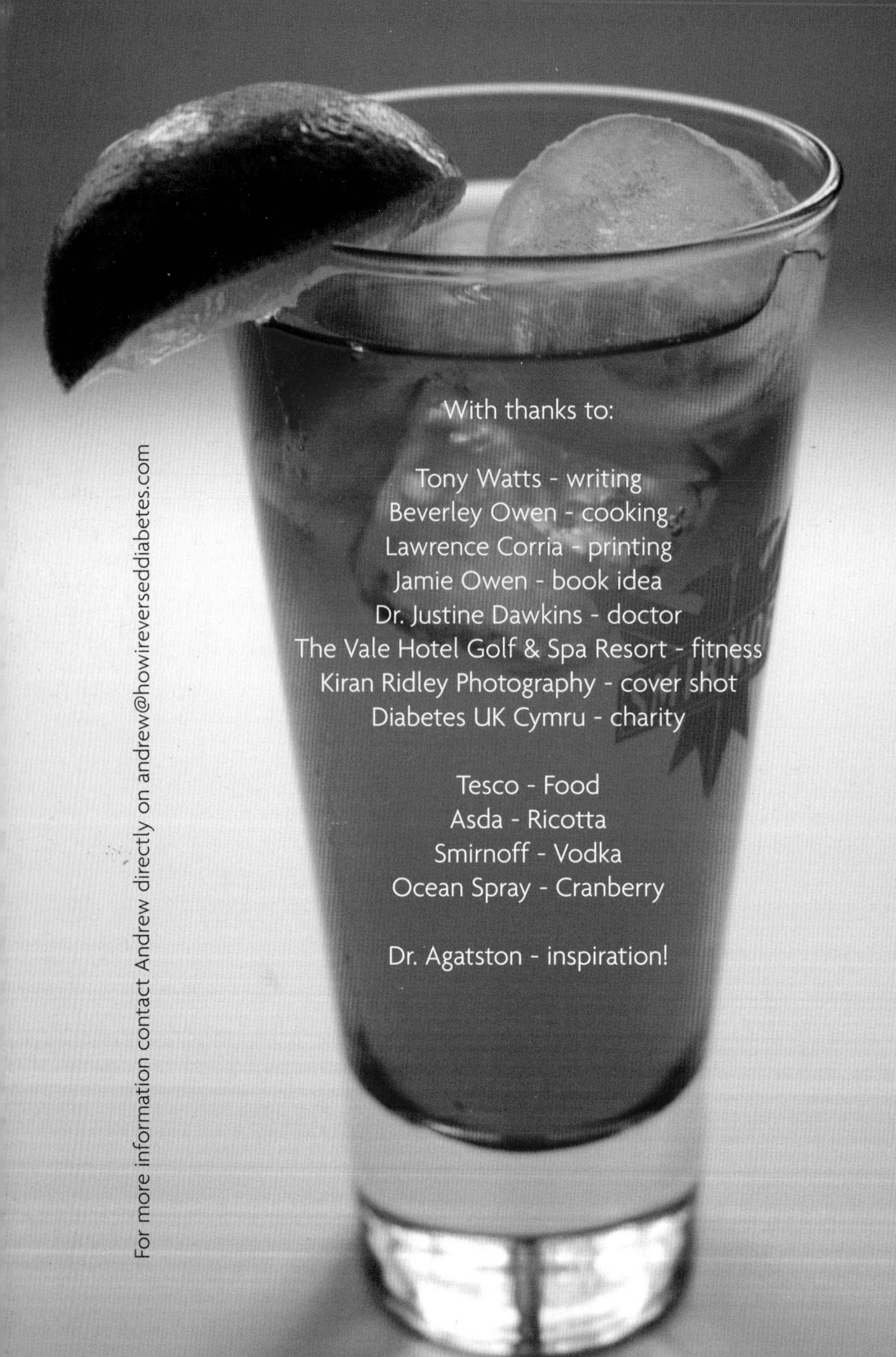

With thanks to:

Tony Watts - writing
Beverley Owen - cooking
Lawrence Corria - printing
Jamie Owen - book idea
Dr. Justine Dawkins - doctor
The Vale Hotel Golf & Spa Resort - fitness
Kiran Ridley Photography - cover shot
Diabetes UK Cymru - charity

Tesco - Food
Asda - Ricotta
Smirnoff - Vodka
Ocean Spray - Cranberry

Dr. Agatston - inspiration!

For more information contact Andrew directly on andrew@howireverseddiabetes.com